The Managed Health Care Dictionary

Second Edition

Richard Rognehaugh
Hospital Administrator
Managed Care Executive

AN ASPEN PUBLICATION®
Aspen Publishers, Inc.
Gaithersburg, Maryland
1998

Library of Congress Cataloging-in-Publication Data

Rognehaugh, Richard.
The managed health care dictionary/Richard Rognehaugh.
—2nd ed.
p. cm.
Includes bibliographical references and index.
ISBN 0-8342-1144-0 (paperback)
1. Managed care plans (Medical care)—Dictionaries.
I. Title.
RA413.R58   1998
362.1′04258′03—dc21
98-3103
CIP

Orders: (800) 638-8437
Customer Service: (800) 234-1660

About Aspen Publishers • For more than 35 years, Aspen has been a leading professional publisher in a variety of disciplines. Aspen's vast information resources are available in both print and electronic formats. We are
committed to providing the highest quality information available in the
most appropriate format for our customers. Visit Aspen's Internet site for
more information resources, directories, articles, and a searchable version
of Aspen's full catalog, including the most recent publications: **http://
www.aspenpub.com**
Aspen Publishers, Inc. • The hallmark of quality in publishing
Member of the worldwide Wolters Kluwer group.

Editorial Services: Kathryn Lynch
Library of Congress Catalog Card Number: 98-3103
ISBN: 0-8342-1144-0

Printed in the United States of America

1 2 3 4 5

Table of Contents

Foreword.. v

Preface... vii

Acknowledgments ix

Using the Dictionary.............................. xi

The Managed Health Care Dictionary 1

Foreword

The Managed Health Care Dictionary will lead to a single resource for patients, physicians, hospital staff, integrated health system employees, trade associations, HCFA and other federal sector agencies, group practices, insurance industry officials, attorneys, the Department of Defense, corporate employers and purchasers of health care coverage, and consultants—all of whom have never had a comprehensive collection of terms outside their arena.

A powerful and affordable addition to any personal or organizational managed care library!

—Peter R. Kongstvedt, MD
Partner, Ernst & Young
Washington, DC
Author of The Managed Health Care Handbook,
Third Edition, *Aspen Publishers, Inc.*

All new fields of human endeavor immediately create a lexicon which isolates all but the cognoscenti. Those of us in the health care field, worn down by our recent struggle with "baud rates," "open architecture databases," and "distributed processing client server" of the electronic revolution are now deluged with the acronyms of "managed care."

Richard Rognehaugh has performed a great service by compiling a reference source which not only defines the mysterious terms but provides a context to make them meaningful.

With the success of our various enterprises in the $900 billion health care industry literally hanging on the thread of our understanding of our options and our contracts, availability of this kind of information is supercritical....

—Jonathan Titus, MD
The "R" Group
Cambridge, Maryland

Preface

The intended audience of *The Managed Health Care Dictionary* is remarkably diverse. This resource addresses terms used across the industry, including health maintenance organizations, preferred provider organizations, physician hospital organizations, individual practice associations, physicians, group practice physicians and staff, patients as policyholders of health insurance, hospitals and hospital integrated systems, and the rising structures of physician management corporations. It also will appeal to students of health care, as well as to managed care executives and their staff, commercial insurers, Medicare, Medicaid, Health Care Financing Administration, state health or insurance regulators or staff, underwriters, actuaries, Information Systems staff, other federal programs such as CHAMPUS and Department of Defense Tricare, and certainly consultants desiring an expanded background.

This book emerged as a result of current literature's shortcoming in not providing a quick reference to supplement the many books on managed care. Although many excellent resources exist, they lack an adequate dictionary capacity or present a single or limited perspective. They often are constructed so that a reader does not recall exactly where to return weeks or months later to get a good definition.

For the first edition and beyond, the goal of this dictionary has been to emerge as the Gold Standard in comprehensive managed care terminology. Just as our world's languages have evolved from simple to complex structures over time, the managed care industry is evolving with contracts that have a spectrum of complex options, despite desires to keep them simple. Our commitment to *The Managed Health Care Dictionary* is to carefully add emerging terms and perspectives in subsequent editions, to remain current within multiple stages of regional managed care markets as they mature.

As readers, we tend to approach any given subject from our current or past perspectives. The dictionary not only will assist you from your perspectives but also will share other perspectives, if they exist. If a term appears to be lengthy, please consider subtle differences within the definition. Other seemingly "non–managed care" terms are listed because of their centrality for contracts specifying coverage minimums, or the type of care to be included. Group practices may have wondered how hospitals or HMOs view the world and may actually catch a better glimpse of their constraints and business motivations through the definitions. If a term leads to another subsequent reference, you may have a new opportunity to perform a critical comparison that has not been previously possible within other narrative publications or periodicals.

Perhaps there have been times when you have wished that a contract negotiation or conference lecture would slow down while you could clarify a term. Yet the pace of the environment simply does not allow for this courtesy. Here, you will find the terms for basic understanding, with the most frequently used words in today's health care contracts, literature, and even political debates. (Try mastering five pages a day!)

If you are pleased that some of these terms are defined from the multiple perspectives of a physician, a hospital, or an insurer—but you feel that there is still a viewpoint missing—please consider joining in our commitment to assemble the industry's premier dictionary. Share your additional definitions or perspectives with Aspen at http://www.aspenpub.com. FAX your comments to (301) 417-7550 or write Aspen Publishers, Inc., 200 Orchard Ridge Drive, Suite 200, Gaithersburg, MD 20878, citing the reference to *The Managed Health Care Dictionary*. Look for subsequent expanded editions in printed and electronic format. We are committed to allowing this resource to meet future needs, and we solicit your feedback to further improve the outcome.

Acknowledgments

The inspiration for this book came from the many patients and health care staff that I have had the privilege to serve in the past 28 years, in hopes of developing a "friendlier" set of definitions for the rapidly expanding area of managed care. Thanks to Jacqulin and Alexis, to Emery Joe and Charlotte Rognehaugh, and to Donald and Geneva Wilson for support along the way. Many thanks to Jack Bruggeman of Aspen Publishers for helping this look easy and to John Brooks for his talent and energy. Finally, thanks to the many leaders, mentors, and colleagues who have shared and guided for the benefit of the patients we are committed to serve.

Using the Dictionary

I. Application

This resource is designed to be either a quick-reference dictionary, a tool to compare and contrast terms, a device to aid in the review of contracts or managed care literature, or a mechanism to further study the field of managed care—aside from a narrative or case study setting. Although there are many books with topical discussions involving current managed care applications, it may be difficult for the reader to quickly return to a specific portion of the book containing a desired term. Also, glossaries are often written with sparse coverage of key terms and may be written only from a single perspective of either a physician, hospital, or payer. This dictionary offers an expanded presentation of terms and definitions from multiple perspectives. Comparative references are given to terms which may be used in "early" or "mature" managed care markets, when applicable; and contrasts with similar terms are pointed out in hopes the reader can gain a better appreciation for either the spectrum of managed care structures or the relationships and evolutions within managed care markets.

II. Arrangement of Terms

Terms are arranged alphabetically.

III. Variations and Synonyms

An effort has been made to link all multiple variations or synonyms to a single term, normally an acronym. The selection of the *primary* acronym, to which the variations or synonyms refer, does not necessarily mean that it is universally the most accepted term but among the most common.

IV. Selection of Primary Acronyms

In cases of multiple variations or synonyms for a single term or in cases where an expanded set of words form an acronym, the definition should be found alongside the acronym. So the expanded set of words will instruct the reader to see the acronym (i.e., for the words *adjusted average per capita cost*, the reader is instructed to find the definition under AAPCC).

V. Terms with the Same Meaning

The forwarding instruction "see AAPCC" means that *adjusted average per capita cost* and *AAPCC* have the same meaning.

VI. Terms Not Having the Same Meaning

The instruction *see also* is used to convey an alternate term, or a term which may help to develop a better understanding of an area or term but is not intended to have the same meaning as the forwarding instruction of *see*. In many cases, a direct comparison within the definition is intended to compare and contrast one term with another.

AAAHC—Accreditation Association for Ambulatory Health Care; originally the Joint Commission's ambulatory review function, before its separate formation in 1979; serves as an accreditation authority for ambulatory health care entities through the formation of standards, performance measurement, consulting, and education as necessary; reviews care quality, QA, clinical records, environmental safety, governance, administration, and professional development; *see also Joint Commission, NCQA, and URAC*

AAHP—American Association of Health Plans; created with the merger of GHAA and AMCRA; announced in February 1996 as the trade association serving nearly 1,000 HMOs, PPOs, and other managed care organizations representing nearly 100 million enrollees in America; *see also AMCRA, and GHAA*

AAPCC—adjusted average per capita cost, used by the Health Care Financing Administration as the calculation for the funds required to care for Medicare recipients; risk contract reimbursement is based on 95% of the AAPCC fee-for-service expenditures on a 5-year rolling average for a county or parish; the 122 AAPCC actuarial stratification includes factors for age, sex, Medicaid eligibility, institutional status, the presence of end-stage renal disease, and whether a person has both Part A and Part B of Medicare; HCFA uses these rates to make monthly payments to contractors that agree to accept risk and treat Medicare patients; the draft 1995 congressional legislation would cap AAPCC updates at a 5.7% average; *see also Medicare risk*

AARP—American Association of Retired Persons; a substantial lobby influence on Medicare managed care legislation, such as MediChoice

abstract—*see discharge summary*

access—generally used to describe the ease of obtaining medical care by the patient; access is measured by the availability of medical services within a format that is convenient to the patient (which may include handicapped provisions, and accommodations for language or sight, as well as the convenience of a location); applications to HCFA for federally qualified HMOs must include a response to "availability, accessibility and continuity of service" including: hours of operation at locations where health care is provided, how the HMO ensures continuity of care for all services, a description of plans for handling members who leave the service area for more than 90 days, and a description of recordkeeping through which pertinent information relating to health care of enrollees is accumulated and is readily available to appropriate professionals

access indicators—*see access measures*

access measures—information that indicates how easy it is for a patient to gain access to medical services, including indicators of timeliness of care, annual turnover of PCPs, patient choice of at least two PCPs, waiting time for urgent care and routine visits, timeliness of test results to patient and physician, availability of physicians and other caregivers, and geographical convenience; one of the key quality indicators for treating disease

access point—there are multiple access points for a patient to enter the continuum of care, each with a corresponding cost and appropriateness; the goal of managed care systems is to educate the patient to use the lowest appropriate access point, and to have that access point available for use, i.e., urgent care or routine care rather than emergency room care

accidental bodily injury—physical injury sustained as the result of an accident

accountable health plan—*see AHP*

Accreditation Association for Ambulatory Health Care—*see AAAHC*

accrual—an HMO establishes an account that holds an amount of money from revenues; this account is designed to cover estimated claim expenses and the lag payment requirements; *see also IBNR, and lag factor*

accumulation period—within the context of deductibles, this is the period of time used (for the contract year) in which the enrollee bears claims costs until the deductible amount is reached; *see also deductible*

ACR—adjusted community rate or rating; a type of rate setting that involves further refinement of rates (beyond that of community rating) by adjusting for key variables within patient groups; mandated by HCFA as the Medicare projection tool to be used by HMOs and CMPs performing Medicare risk; this rate, which allows for a typical percent of profit, is the result of adjusting other, more specific group plan data so that the rating more closely approximates the type of utilization that would be experienced by Medicare enrollees (as opposed to experience rating, for example, which would give actual costs for a known group of enrollees); *see also community rating, and experience rating*

actively-at-work—because much of the current health coverage still is based on employment status, this phrase is used within many contracts to indicate that an employee is working on the day the policy goes into effect, or medical coverage will not be provided until that employee returns to work; for other relationships of employment status to coverage; *see also continuation, conversion privilege, disenrollment, and extension of benefits*

Activities of Daily Living—*see ADL*

actual charge—physician's actual fee for service at the time the insurance claim is submitted to the insurance company, government payer, or HMO; *see also FFS*

actuarial assumptions—the assumptions that an actuary uses in calculating the expected costs and revenues of the plan; examples include utilization rates, age and sex mix of enrollees, disability level distribution of the population, and cost for medical services

actuarial factors—term used by HCFA to mean actuarial assumptions; *see actuarial assumptions*

actuary—an employee within the insurance industry or related field who is trained and recognized as an accredited insurance mathematician to calculate premium rates, reserves, and dividends within a given plan; and prepares statistical studies, reports, and projections based on the experience of given populations or plans

acute care—the class of medical service that deals with needs that are expected to be of short duration (30 days or less); services primarily oriented toward medical problems that require intensive attention and treatment to restore a previous state of health or prevent the worsening of a present state; the goal of acute care programs is to provide access within a maximum time limit, such as 24 hours; most commonly found in hospitals, surgical centers, and clinics; *see also continuum of care, and postacute care*

additional benefits to Medicare risk—one of the most attractive features of managed care to Medicare beneficiaries who seek comprehensive, quality care for the least out-of-pocket expense and least amount of paperwork is for Risk HMOs and CMPs to offer additional benefits; in a recent HCFA report from the Operations & Oversight Team of the Office of Managed Care, the numbers of the 154 HMOs contracting with HCFA offering additional benefits are listed as: routine physicals (131), eye exams (121), immunizations (116), ear exams (100), outpatient drugs (65), dental (48), foot care (46), health education (34), lenses (7), and hearing aids (5)

additional drug benefit list—pharmaceuticals that are typically of long-term or chronic usage that are approved by a commercial plan or federal entity, commonly undergoing an annual review for completeness and appropriateness; objectives of this list are to clearly establish the most effective drugs, with the lowest cost when multiple drugs may be candidates, as well as to have a standardized list approved in advance for patient convenience; *see also formulary*

adjudication—review of claims to determine payment; for claims involving appeal, adjudication leads to a final determination of payment action or judgment

adjusted average per capita cost—*see AAPCC*

adjusted community rate or rating—*see ACR*

adjustment to payment—if the HMO's or CMP's actual number of enrollees in each class differs from the number of estimated enrollees for the purposes of determining advance payments, an adjustment is made in subsequent months to account for these changes

ADL—Activities of Daily Living; used to describe the basic personal activities as standards for a patient to perform independently of home health, nursing assistance, or more intensive health services, i.e., cooking, bathing, dressing, or obtaining necessary personal or public transportation

administration loading—*see administrative costs*

administrative costs—dollar amount that is in excess of the prospective actuarial cost for health care services; costs including services associated with payment of claims, enrollment, marketing, or overhead; prospectively paid premiums by enrollees minus capitated payments to physicians results in the value or percentage of administrative costs; *see also ASO*

administrative services only—*see ASO*

admission certification—used as a more precise term than admission review or concurrent review, to indicate similar activities, but those activities that are also certified by a utilization review committee to ensure that criteria are met for admission

admission education—*see preadmission education*

admission placement center—a centralized function to provide consultation for physicians within a hospital or plan, regarding the lowest cost treatment alternatives that are appropriate for the patient; physicians may gain telephone or direct personal access to the placement center staff, in order to maximize use of a continuum of care as options to acute admission; the savings that result from efficient care placement may be shared with physicians through a bonus arrangement; *see also continuum of care, and PCR*

admission review—review for appropriateness and medical necessity of admission; *see also medically necessary*

admissions per thousand—*see APT*

admits—the quantity of inpatient admissions to any type of inpatient facility

admitting privilege—the basic authorization for a provider to admit a patient to an inpatient hospital or surgical setting, based on approval by a medical or hospital board after review of the provider's license, training, and formal education; *see also PAC*

ADS—*see alternate delivery system*

adult day care—an emerging element of geriatric care services, directed toward a multiple of lower cost options for seniors, to include a mix of nursing care, therapy services, group day settings, rehabilitation, and home health care services, which enable key staff, such as a community health nurse, to see more patients in a day (from 6–8 to 12–14); not traditionally covered under Medicare, but may hold promise for Medicare and Medicaid managed care; *see also adult day health care center*

adult day health care center—a care setting that combines adult day care with more advanced health services that are provided by members of a licensed health staff, enabling the center to accommodate adult patients that have medical needs beyond adult day care

advanced directive—the policy, and implementation of policy, to offer each patient the opportunity to complete a living will prior to admission; required by Medicare for admission, and also a required part of the enrollment and marketing literature that must be received by all Medicare risk HMO enrollees

adverse selection—a phenomenon that occurs within the mix of covered lives for a plan, when patients with high health care utilization habits select a particular plan, in greater numbers than are otherwise representative of the population as a whole; *see also favorable selection, and risk adjustment*

advice nurse—the use of a registered nurse to answer questions for patients who need to make a decision regarding their care, or the care of a family member; a utilization management strategy to reduce the demand for physician visits by providing telephonic advice through a nurse; advice nurse programs generally err on the side of recommending that the patient should see a physician, rather than to chance missing a condition that may be more serious than what appears to be conveyed on the telephone

advocate—*see patient advocate*

AFDC—Aid to Families with Dependent Children program; established by the Social Security Act of 1935 to give cash payments to children and their caretakers who need support due to the death, disablement, or continuous absence or unemployment of one or more parent from the home; thresholds are governed by state criteria

affiliated health care provider—any hospital, clinic, outpatient services facility, individual physician, or surgeon listed under the definition of provider, or groups of physicians or surgeons that or who may be affiliated with a particular insurer and that by contract provide professional health care services to patients and others in support of the mission and stated initiatives of the named insurer; *see also participating provider*

aftercare—the type of health care services that are sequentially provided after some period of hospitalization or rehabilitation, which are administered based on each patient's condition, with the objective of improving or restoring health to the degree that aftercare is no longer needed; may include any or multiple continuum options under postacute care; *see also postacute care*

age limits—stated maximum and minimum ages that govern eligibility according to health plan contracts

age-at-issuance rating—a health care premium methodology that sets premium levels based on the age of individuals when they first received insurance for health

age-attained rating—a health care premium methodology that sets premium levels based on the current age of the individual requesting insurance

age/sex factor—within the discipline of health care insurance underwriting, this factor accounts for the age and sex risk of medical costs for a given population, with regard to the likely medical claims or health care utilization from such a group

age/sex rate—*see ASR*

Agency for Health Care Policy and Research—*see AHCPR*

aggregate indemnity—the maximum dollar amount that may be collected for any disability or period of disability under an insurance policy

aging report—the report that documents the cycle time for claims processing, or turnaround time for other functions such as adjustments, correspondence, appeals, and grievances; *see also cycle time, and TAT*

AGPA—American Group Practice Association; formed in 1989 to begin a project in outcomes measurement; organized to help insurers, providers, and patients make informed decisions about their health by means of various measurement data on health

AHA—American Hospital Association; a trade association for hospitals

AHCPR—Agency for Health Care Policy and Research; created by Congress in 1989 under Public Law 101-239 as a public health service agency to collect and share information to improve health care delivery, as the successor for the National Center for Health Services Research (NCHSR); AHCPR is not a regulator such as the FDA or HCFA, but promotes biomedical and health services research of public benefit, with over 30 projects related to managed care plans, networks, quality, and accountability; charged with enhancing the quality, appropriateness, and effectiveness of health care services and access to these services

AHP—Accountable Health Plan; *see managed health care plan*

AHSR—Association for Health Services Research; a national membership organization formed exclusively to promote the field of health services research and to strengthen the relationship between the users and producers of health research

Aid to Families with Dependent Children—*see AFDC*

AIDS—acquired immune deficiency syndrome, a disease caused by a virus that damages the body's immune system, thereby destroying its ability to fight off illness; some plans provide a carve out for treatment of AIDS patients; *see also carve out, and chronic care capitation*

alignment of incentives—a phrase used to describe the relatively new economic arrangements of sharing between physicians and hospitals that creates an incentive for physicians to accept capitation

allied health personnel—*see midlevel practitioner*

allocated benefits—medical claims for services and supplies are collected against individual or group allocated benefits, subject to any maximum amounts payable under terms of the contract

allowable charge—amount that CHAMPUS determines as the reasonable fee for a service, and on which CHAMPUS figures the patient's cost-share for covered care; based on 75% to 80% of the allowable charge, depending on whether the patient is the dependent of active duty, a retiree, or dependent of retiree; charges for supplies or services that meet the criteria of covered expenses

allowable cost—from the context of a federally qualified HMO— the direct and indirect costs, including normal standby costs incurred, that are proper and necessary for efficient delivery of needed health care services, including provider costs, and costs for marketing, enrollment, membership, and operation of the HMO, that are peculiar to health care prepayment organizations; *see also allowable charge*

allowance for contractual deductions—an accounting mechanism used by hospitals that works to demonstrate the difference between the actual hospital charges for health care services in a given accounting period and the influence of contractual negotiated payment discounts by third party payers for these same services

allowance for uncollectibles—in health care finance, subtracting from the gross operating revenue the reduction in revenue due to serving medically indigent patients and courtesy allowances; may also include all bad debt service

all-payer rate setting—the system within Maryland, as of 1993, designed to contain costs by establishing maximum target rates for doctors (not applicable when a physician's rate is below the target), through an appointed committee, and hospital rates for Medicaid, Medicare, and commercial payers; an FFS system in Minnesota was repealed before implementation in 1995, and another 1993 law in Florida

ALOS—average length of stay; calculated as the average number of patient days of hospitalization for each admission, expressed as an average of the population within the plan for a given period of time

alternate delivery system—any health care beyond the traditional private practice fee for service; provision of health services in settings that are often more cost-effective than an inpatient, acute care hospital, such as skilled and intermediary nursing facilities, hospice programs, and in-home services; alternate delivery systems may include IPAs, PPOs, and HMOs

AMA—American Medical Association, a national professional society of physicians

ambulatory care—health care services that are rendered on an outpatient basis, or to patients who are not confined overnight in a health care institution; outpatient care; may be provided within a doctor's office, a medical clinic, acute hospital, or freestanding ambulatory surgery center

ambulatory care center, free-standing—facility with an organized professional staff that provides various medical treatments on an outpatient basis only and that may be one of three types of center, depending on the level of care it is equipped to provide: freestanding emergency center, freestanding urgent care center, or primary care center

ambulatory care review—all outpatient services are reviewed retrospectively to ensure the appropriate utilization of health services

ambulatory patient group—*see APG*

ambulatory setting—the environment for providing health care services that is consistent with the definition of ambulatory care, and may also include mobile units supporting mammography, MRI, or fixed facility locations that provide same day surgery

ambulatory surgery center—*see ASC*

ambulatory utilization review—with the shift of patient care settings from inpatient to outpatient, and the fact that many patients enrolled in managed care plans rarely experience hospitalization, a greater emphasis is required to analyze the care within the ambulatory setting; *see UR*

ambulatory weighted unit—*see relative weighted product*

AMCRA—American Managed Care and Review Association; merged with GHAA (Group Health Association of America, representing large staff and group model HMOs) in 1995; a trade association representing IPA model HMOs, PPOs, and UROs; the new organization is named the American Association of Health Plans; *see also AAHP*

amendment—formal document changing the provisions of an insurance or HMO contract and signed jointly by authorized representatives of the insurer, policyholder, provider, or selected entity

American Association of Health Plans—*see AAHP*

AMGA—American Medical Group Association; consists of 350 group practices, PPOs, and IPAs, based in Alexandria, Virginia; active support for their members, including an interest in easing antitrust regulation that would result in IPAs and PPOs being able to compete with managed care plans; *see also PSN*

ancillary—outpatient or auxiliary services to support diagnostic workup of the patient, or supplemental services needed as part of providing other care; ancillary services include anesthesia, lab, radiology, or pharmacy; other than room, board, medical, and nursing services

ancillary charge—the billing and collection of ancillary services are sometimes handled as additional services performed, such as laboratory procedures, radiology, anesthesia, or pharmacy charges (which may exceed the plan's maximum allowable)

ancillary provider—various contracts include a definition for ancillary provider, which would include any individual or corporation, partnership, or other legal entity recognized under law to provide home health, hospice, skilled nursing facility, or other such services; also, the ancillary provider must have the power under its own organizational charter to commit its provider members by contract

ancillary services—*see ancillary*

anniversary—the beginning of a subscriber or group's benefit year

annual adjustment—a contract provision that gives either party, such as an insurer and provider, the opportunity to review payment rates or business volume, in terms of the appropriateness of extending the contract under existing terms

annual deductible—*see deductible*

antikickback statute—forbids referral kickback remuneration of any kind for Medicare and Medicaid, imposing criminal sanctions; kickbacks cannot be solicited, taken, or offered for business involving the purchase or lease of health care goods or services; procurements of physician practices by hospitals are reviewed by the Office of the Inspector General in terms of anything that can be considered referral payments of a continuing nature, i.e., good will, noncompete clauses, and the amount and manner of compensation; *see also Stark I, and Stark II*

anti–managed care legislation—the name given to an increasing number of state legislative or regulatory proposals that are considered by some to be unfriendly to managed care, such as any willing provider, maternity length of stay, or patient protection act; *see also any willing provider, maternity length of stay legislation, and PPA (patient protection act)*

antitrust exemption law—*see state action immunity*

antitrust laws—related to the health care industry by preventing monopolies, price fixing, or restrictive trade within markets or regions; *see also Clayton Act, COPA law, FTC Act, and Sherman Act*

any willing provider—*see AWP laws; see also exclusivity*

APG—ambulatory patient groups; a modification of ambulatory visit groups (AVGs), developed as an outpatient classification scheme for HCFA; APGs are the reimbursement methodology for outpatient procedures as DRGs are for inpatient days; APGs provide for a fixed reimbursement to an institution for outpatient procedures or visits and incorporate data regarding the reason for the visit and patient data; they prevent unbundling of ancillary services

appeals and hearings—a plan must outline its procedures to handle member appeals and hearings; Medicare applicants seeking status as federally qualified HMOs will include these procedures in the Documents section, including when these procedures will be applied in place of the member grievance procedure

application—statement of relevant facts signed by an individual who is seeking insurance or by a prospective group policyholder; the application is the basis for the insurer's decision to issue a policy; the application usually is incorporated into the policy

application integrator—software that is used between different managed care applications to provide data conversion and transmission without the need for special programming to interface two or more applications, thereby reducing the cost of systems interface

appropriateness measures—indicators that show discrepancies between the actual care given and the level of care that is considered "necessary," thereby representing the plan's ability to provide cost-effective care; one of the quality indicators associated with the treatment of disease

approval—approval by a utilization review function or authority to provide a service; approval by a state insurance department regarding the filing application of policy and certificate forms and rates of a plan; underwriting approval signifies the insurer's acceptance of the risk outlined in the application; policy approval by an officer of an insurer signifies the acceptance of an offer from an applicant or policyholder in the form of a contract for new insurance

approved charge—Medicare's ceiling within a geographical area for a particular covered benefit

approved health care facility—as governed by an accrediting agency such as the Joint Commission, or after receiving a Certificate of Need or other mechanism to license, certify, or authorize the provision of health care under state law

APR—adjusted payment rate; the amount of money that HCFA pays to risk contract HMOs; the figure is derived from the county AAPCC for the service area adjusted for the relative risks of the plan's enrollees; *see also AAPCC*

APT—admissions per thousand; the number of hospital admissions per 1,000 health plan members; derived by the number of admissions/member months, times 1,000 members, times the number of months within the time period being analyzed

arbitrage—*see capitation arbitrage*

arbitration—in the event of dispute or difference in opinion arising out of agreements between certain plans and reinsurers, or between other entities, the parties typically agree that such disputes will be submitted to and settled by arbitration in accordance with an authority such as the Bermuda Arbitration Act of 1986, which is considered to be the sole means by which disputes will be resolved

ASC—ambulatory surgery center; performs surgery of an uncomplicated nature that has traditionally been done in the more expensive inpatient setting but can be done with equal efficiency without hospital admission; centers may be hospital-based, sponsored, or independently owned in competition with hospitals; also called same day surgery center

ASO—administrative services only, typically a portion of the per member per month rate that is performed either by a payer or provider; a contract between an insurance company and a self-funded plan where the insurance company performs administrative services only and does not assume any risk; services usually include claims processing but may include other services such as actuarial analysis or utilization review; *see also ERISA*

ASR—age/sex rate; the methodology used to develop health insurance premium pricing and group billing rates for various groupings of age and sex, using the applicable age/sex factors for a particular insurance product or group of patients; reflects the demographics of a group, rather than charging a premium for a single patient or family; *see also age/sex factor*

asset merger model—a legal model for mature market integrated health care systems, involving a single governance body of one board and one CEO, single ownership, single identity and name; also called full network ownership; *see also holding company legal model*

assignment of benefits—the payment of medical benefits directly to a provider of care rather than to a member; generally requires either a contract between the health plan and the provider, or a written release from the subscriber to the provider allowing the provider to bill the health plan; the transfer of one's interest or policy benefits to another party

assisted living center—a relatively new component of the health care setting requiring the least amount of medical care as an option that provides more independence than nursing home care, and yet provides the safeguards not available to a patient living alone; daily support such as nutritious meal preparation or minimal medical assistance such as IV therapy is often the only care needed

Association for Health Services Research—*see AHSR*

association group—a group formed from members of a trade or professional association for group insurance under one master health insurance contract

assumption of financial risk—the risk an HMO bears on behalf of its members; according to CFR-42, each HMO must assume full financial risk on a prospective basis for the provision of basic health services, except that it may obtain insurance or make other arrangements to cover the following: for the cost of providing an aggregate value of more than $5,000 to an enrollee in any year; the cost of legitimate out-of-area care; for not more than 90% of the amount by which its costs for any fiscal year exceed 115% of its income; and to cover risk for its participating providers

assumption of risk—in this case, the specific knowledge of a person who knowingly pursues a course after being advised of the dangers, and still consents to medical treatment, thereby becoming ineligible to sue for damages unless there has been some other malpractice

ATM—asynchronous transfer mode; a method of high-speed data transmission to support local area networks (LANs), metropolitan area networks (MANs), or wide area networks (WANs) by compressing information for data, voice, and visual systems

at-risk contracting—a managed care strategy that involves the assumption of financial risk to some degree or percentage, for some portion of a given patient population; *see also risk, risk corridor, and risk HMOs/CMPs*

attachment point—*see point of attachment*

attending physician—the physician responsible for the care and treatment of a patient in the hospital; a consulting physician or a physician employed by the hospital is not the attending physician

attrition rate—disenrollment expressed as a percentage of total membership; a plan with 40,000 members with a 2% attrition rate would need to gain 800 new members each month to retain the initial 40,000 covered lives

audit adjustment report—a statement by Medicare auditors of their proposed changes in costs claimed by the provider in its cost report

audit of provider treatment—*see provider audit*

authorization—the approval by a primary care provider in order for plan coverage to be granted for hospitalization or certain procedures; approval from the health plan for procedures or hospitalization

authorized provider—doctor or other individual authorized to provide care or a hospital or supplier approved by CHAMPUS to provide medical care and supplies

availability—*see access*

average cost per claim—a financial amount, representing the sum of the medical charge and administrative charge for services provided within the categories of admissions, physician services, and outpatient claims

average length of stay—*see ALOS*

average wholesale price—*see AWP*

AVGs—ambulatory visit groups are an outpatient classification scheme of 571 groupings

AWP—average wholesale price; the standard charge for a pharmacy item; derived by taking the average cost of the item to a pharmacy as charged by a large representation of pharmacy wholesale suppliers (for items not otherwise being sold at a discount)

AWP laws—any willing provider laws; requires managed care organizations to grant network enrollment to any provider who is willing to join, as long as they meet provisions outlined in the plan; the central issue is the fairness of physician deselection by a plan, and conversely the plan's ability to reduce medical costs by eliminating overuse of physicians; multiple state laws challenge and establish policy

B

back office function—generally refers to the administrative services, or some components of member services, physician services, accounting, and claims reimbursement, that must be performed in support of managed care contracting by either an insurer, MSO, PHO, TPA; a managed care entity makes a determination of whether it is willing or able to perform these functions as an essential core business for a profit, or whether it is better to outsource the functions

backward integration—the strategy or activity of a company that wishes to enter or expand its presence within a market, in which it seeks to purchase or merge with others who precede its designated set of services

balance billing—the practice of a provider billing a patient for all charges not paid for by the insurance plan, because those charges are above the plan's UCR (usual, customary, and reasonable) practice or may be considered medically unnecessary; plans are increasingly prohibiting providers from balance billing except for allowed copays, coinsurance, and deductibles

Balanced Budget Act of 1997—Title IV of this act includes provisions for Medicare, Medicaid, and children's health and amendments to existing legislation that allowed for establishment of the Medicare+Choice plan, special rules for Medical Savings Accounts, a Medicare subvention demonstration project for military retirees, the addition of high-deductible Medigap policies, broad health prevention measures, and rural health initiatives; *see also Medicare+Choice*

bargaining representative—within the context of employee health benefit plans, a bargaining representative is an individual or entity designated or selected, under any applicable federal, state, or local law, or public entity collective bargaining agreement, to represent employees in collective bargaining, or any other employee representative designated or selected under any law

base capitation—the amount of money that is required to cover the cost of care for the average enrollee, minus any carve outs for mental health, pharmacy, and such (plans differ widely on the basic inclusions)

basic care—the level of services required to maintain a nursing home resident's activities of daily living; includes personal care, ambulation, supervision, and safety; this care can be provided by a nurse aide, practical nurse, or a family member

basic health services—benefits that all federally qualified HMOs must offer, defined under subpart A, 417.104(a) of the Federal HMO Regulations, to include at least: physician services, outpatient services to include diagnostics, inpatient services, instructions on how to secure emergency care in and out of the service area, 20 outpatient visits per enrollee per year, home health, and preventive services

batch—a group of claims for different patients from one office submitted in one computer transmission; or a group of claims processed by a claims processor

BC/BS—Blue Cross/Blue Shield

bed days per 1,000—*see days per thousand*

behavioral offset—*see volume offset*

benchmarking—a process of comparing one's own health care practice or entity to the finest in the business, in order to improve the quality of care or services by constantly observing how the most efficient comparable organizations across the country are run; some accreditation organizations, such as the Joint Commission, have adopted Malcolm Baldridge formats and have made benchmarking an essential element for planning within health care organizations; *see also QI*

beneficiary—person or persons specified by a policyholder as eligible to receive insurance policy proceeds (private or government)

beneficiary liability—may be funds required from the beneficiary to the plan in the form of premiums, deductibles, or copay amounts, or for services not covered in the plan

benefit—amount payable by the insurance company to a claimant, assignee, or beneficiary when the insured suffers a loss covered by the policy

benefit design—a process of determining what level of coverage or type of service should be included within a health plan or specific product, at specified rates of reimbursement, based on a multiple of relatively unstandardized and often unique factors, such as market pressure, cost, clinical effectiveness and medical evidence, legislated mandate, medical necessity, and preventive value; *see also covered services*

benefit levels—the degree to which a person is entitled to receive services based on his/her contract with a plan or insurer

benefit package—*see covered services; see also standard benefit package*

benefit payment schedule—*see covered services*

benefit plan—*see covered services*

benefit stabilization fund—similar to a withhold or pool but with a specific application for Medicare risk; used to describe a fund established by HCFA at the request of an HMO or CMP with a new risk contract to withhold a portion of the per capita payments, for payment in a subsequent contract period for the purpose of stabilizing fluctuations in the availability of the additional benefits provided by the HMO or CMP to its Medicare enrollees

best practice protocol—*see medical protocols*

biased selection—*see risk selection*

bifurcated structure—often the title given to health care insurance coverage that has a separation between the system for hospital expenses, and the system for medical coverage, as in the early structures of Blue Cross for hospital care and Blue Shield for surgical and other medical charges; *see also Blue Cross plan, and Blue Shield*

bilateral exclusives—*see two-way exclusives*

billed charge—*see submitted charge; see also FFS*

billed charges with maximum—the hospital and HMO agree that the HMO will pay billed charges, but a ceiling or cap is placed on charges, with the HMO responsible for all charges up to the cap

billed claims—*see submitted charge; see also FFS*

blanket contract—contract of health insurance that covers a class of persons not individually identified; used for groups such as athletic teams and for employee travel policies

blanket medical expense—a provision that entitles the insured person to collect up to a maximum established in the policy for all hospital and medical expenses incurred, without any limitations on individual types of medical expenses

blended capitation—a reimbursement mechanism that mixes some proportion of traditional fee for service with some proportion of AAPCC capitated reimbursement; blended capitation is encouraged for use within the Medicare Choices demonstration project

blended per diem—*see hybrid per diem*

block grant—commonly used to describe federal funds provided to the state level as a nucleus of support for Medicaid provisions by the state to its beneficiaries; *see also MediGrant*

block grant—county level—the passing of Medicaid funds from the state level to the county level, to be spent either as the county deems appropriate, or with certain limits; the governor of New York proposed block grants to the county level in New York's fiscal 1997 budget

Blue Cross—nonprofit membership corporation providing protection against the cost of hospital care in a limited geographic area; in some cases protects against the costs of surgical and professional care

Blue Cross Association (BCA)—the national nonprofit organization to which the 70 Blue Cross plans in the United States voluntarily belong; BCA administers programs of licensure and approval for Blue Cross plans, provides specific services related to the writing and administering of health care benefits across the country and represents the Blue Cross plans in national affairs; an organization founded to promote the betterment of public health and security; to secure the widest public acceptance of voluntary nonprofit prepayment of health services; and to provide national services to local Blue Cross and Blue Shield plans; contracts with the federal government as an administrative agency for federal health programs; sponsors and conducts programs on health care and prepayment issues; under contract with the Social Security Administration, BCA is intermediary in the Medicare program for 77% of the participating providers (90% of hospitals, 50% of SNFs, and 76% of home health participants)

Blue Cross plan—formerly tax exempt until 1986, a prepayment organization providing coverage for health care and related services distinguished from the national association, the Blue Cross Association; largely the creation of the hospital industry, it was designed to provide hospitals with a stable source of revenues, although formal association between Blue Cross and the AHA ended in 1972; there are 70 plans in the United States, most of which are regulated by state insurance commissioners under special enabling legislation

Blue Shield—nonprofit membership corporation providing protection against the cost of surgery and other items of medical care in a limited geographic area; some policies also cover hospital care

Blue Shield plan—a plan originally established in 1939 that provides coverage of physician services; the individual plans should be distinguished from the national association of Blue Shield Plans; the relationship between Blue Cross and Blue Shield plans has been cooperative, with the two organizations having a common board, one management, and administered side by side

Blues—also called "the Blues"; the name given to include any or all types of various Blue Cross and Blue Shield medical coverage plans; now represent a shrinking portion of overall health care coverage versus the growing for-profit HMOs

BMAD—Part B Medicare Annual Data Files; contain cost and utilization source data for Medicare Part B; *see also Medicare Part B*

board certified—a physician or other health professional who has passed an exam from a medical specialty board and is thereby certified to provide care within that specialty

board eligible—some health plans describe the caliber of their participating providers in terms of the percentage that are eligible to take the specialty board exam (versus the number who have actually passed the exam—or are board certified), as graduates from an approved medical college or university after completion of the required training and practical experience

bodily injury—injury to the human body, disease or illness sustained by any person, including death at any time resulting from the injury

bonding—an insurance contract by which, in return for a stated fee, a bonding agency guarantees payment of a certain sum to an employer in the event of a financial loss to the employer by the act of a specified employee or by some contingency over which the employer has no control

bonus pool—another term for physician contingency reserve; *see PCR*

brand name identification—any marketing or licensing effort that leads to a strengthened association between consumers of health care services and providers or insurers, directed toward enhancing a purchasing decision of a particular brand by the consumer; may involve making a health care entity's presence better known to gain market share, or a provider's market entry as an HMO by establishing or leasing an HMO license, or marketing a Physician Directory extensively through newspaper, radio, or television in order to direct patients to a particular PHO's providers

break-even point—the number of covered lives necessary for a plan or provider to reach an equal position between costs and revenue, at any given time

broad panel health plan—an inclusive network of a fairly large number of hospitals and physician groups within an insurer's health plan, versus an exclusive network; the HMO specifically attempts to build the widest possible network in order to not exclude employers' or patients' favorite providers, as long as the providers have acceptable practice performance and utilization; *see also exclusion, and exclusivity*

broadly representative enrollment—under HCFA guidelines, each HMO must offer enrollment to persons who are broadly representative of the various age, social, and income groups within its service area; not more than 75% of enrollees may be from the medically underserved population unless the area is rural

broker—person licensed by the state who places business with several insurers; *see also patient broker*

broker channeling—*see patient broker channeling incentive*

budget neutral—within the context of current legislation for Medicare, payment rates will be adjusted to ensure that total spending under the new rules will remain constant

buffing—the practice of one physician transferring a known or potentially high-cost patient to another physician within a managed care environment, rather than see profits eroded

bundled case rate—a single charge or reimbursement mechanism that includes the institutional and professional charges

bundled payment—one payment for a group of related health care treatment and/or services

business coalition—a formation of local, regional, or state business entities for the purpose of influencing health care to bring cost savings, benefit their employees' access or quality of care; may include purchasing alliance negotiations, lobbying for policy reform, or developing common standards; some state-level coalitions include hospitals, IDNs, insurers, trade associations, and others who share the coalition's objectives; *see also purchasing alliance*

C

cafeteria plan—a plan that allows employees to "pick and choose" among two or more benefits, in which an employer can provide employees with a choice of taxable or nontaxable benefits and employees are taxed only to the extent of the value of the taxable benefit chosen; may include accident or health insurance, and dependent care assistance; if a benefit is chosen by an employee in agreement for a voluntary salary reduction, then the amount of the salary reduction is considered earned income for the purposes of earned income credit

calendar year—January 1st through December 31st; used as the basis for establishing payment of deductibles to a plan by an enrollee for major medical or PPO, HMO coverage, or in separate provisions for hospital, surgical, and medical plans

call screen transfer capability—allows a telephone call to be transferred, together with a visual set of data about the caller, therefore eliminating the need for asking the caller duplicate questions; a preferred customer service feature, which adds a caring perspective together with response time efficiency; *see also integrated call management*

CalPERS—the California Public Employee Retirement System; a large employee group of nearly 950,000, a huge amount of business for nearly 15 California HMOs; CalPERS represents a type of pioneer experience in negotiating a 5% premium decline in 1995; *see also cost compression*

cap rate—*see capitation rate*

capitated payment—a contractually agreed fee (monthly, bimonthly, or annual) paid by an HMO or CMP to either an IDN, hospital, physician, or group practice, in exchange for health care services to enrolled members

capitation (cap)—the primary reimbursement characteristic of managed care, in which a provider is responsible for treating a population of patients for a prepaid payment arrangement on a per-member basis with no relationship to the amount of care actually received, versus receiving payment for fee-for-service care to an individual patient; a set amount of money received or paid out, based on a prepaid agreement rather than on actual cost of separate episodes of care and services delivered, usually is expressed in units of per-member-per-month (PMPM); may be varied by such factors as age and sex and benefit plan of the enrolled member; *see also FFS, hospital capitation, and prepaid health plan*

capitation arbitrage—in the early stages of capitation within phases of managed care maturity for a given marketplace, an initial advantage of capitation arbitrage goes to the first physician groups, hospitals, or integrated delivery systems that learn to provide managed care efficiently; i.e., if the PMPM pricing equivalent was $50 before any market changes, and a "pioneering" group can bid the care at $38 with costs of only $30, they will be attractive to payers for large patient volumes under capitation—still able to make money before any further cost compression occurs; soon other competitors will duplicate the pricing, and pricing gets very close to cost, hence the arbitrage disappears; *see cost compression, and PMPM*

capitation list—a list that documents the members for whom a capitated payment was received, including any retroactive additions and retroactive deletions; *see also retro add, and retro delete*

capitation rate—providers and HMOs (and other "customer-supplier" entities) negotiate a rate per enrollee, per time period (often monthly); the provider renders all contracted care and services to members for a prospective payment with retroactive adjustments, taking the risk that the capitation rate will be sufficient to cover all of the costs of care to members; similar agreements can be made between the hospital/delivery system, and physician groups, for either PCPs or specialists; *see also capitated payment, and PMPM*

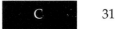

capped entitlement—proposed Democratic plan that features continued federal entitlements for pregnant women, children, the elderly, and disabled, but states would receive a capped amount per beneficiary

captive domicile—captive insurer or reinsurer entities are organized in domiciles (nine states and three territories in the United States among them) that have passed special legislation to foster the formation of captives and promote their benefits to the worldwide risk management community; captives are formed throughout the world and the choice of a captive's domicile may have either little or considerable bearing on the parent entity's risk management program, depending upon tax, reinsurance, administration, and related issues; at the end of 1994 the following top-10 domiciles represented over 70% of the world's existing captives: Bermuda (1,357 total licenses), Cayman Islands (361), Vermont (311), Guernsey (280), Barbados (276), Luxembourg (204), Isle of Man (141), Dublin (114), Singapore (49), and Hawaii (41)

captive enrollment broker—*see patient broker*

captive insurer—underwrites the risk of its parent corporation and affiliates, and insures retained earning to the benefit of the captive's ultimate owner or owners; a subsidiary or affiliate of a hospital or system that is formed to provide professional or other liability coverage on a self-insured basis as an alternative to procuring other commercial insurance

captive management firm—an accounting firm that serves as the home office of a captive insurer, providing directors for the captive board; creating periodic accounts and financial reports; managing the banking, payables, and receivables; serving as Principal Representative; and assisting with audits (most commonly located in Bermuda because of laws more receptive to broad exposure and the ratio of premium underwritings to surplus—the most successful U.S. domicile is Vermont)

captive patient broker—*see patient broker*

care continuum—*see continuum of care*

care coordinator—an individual, typically a PCP or physician extender, who acts as the patient's representative to ensure that appropriate and timely health care is provided, yet with cost-effective utilization; *see also gatekeeper model*

care management system—*see CMS*

care system model—a type of advanced health insurance purchasing cooperative (HIPC) system that includes a virtual market care system for employees with broad choice in plans that do business with the coalition; the coalition has a central purchasing role for employees or consumers; the model includes a coalition entity, provider systems, primary care providers (often in exclusive relationships with providers), and specialist physicians serving multiple providers—and excludes insurers and employers that are present in HIPCs; also called a virtual health plan because of the array of options available for consumer selection; providers that meet coalition criteria are included, which allows employee choice of basic covered services normally covered by employer contribution, or premium services available for out-of-pocket; *see also direct contracting, employer contribution, HIPC, PSN, and purchasing alliance*

carrier—also called payer or payor; a voluntary association, corporation, partnership, or other organization that is engaged in providing, paying for, or reimbursing all or part of the cost of health benefits under group insurance policies or contracts, medical or hospital service agreements, enrollment or subscription contracts, or similar group arrangements, in consideration of premiums or other periodic charges payable to the carrier; an insurer that underwrites policies, administers claims, and in some cases, provides services directly; for Medicare, an entity that contracts with HCFA to process claims for Part B

carrier replacement—*see CR*

carve out—within a capitation environment, a type of service not included as an agreed service to be provided within the con-

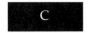

tract, therefore carved out within the PMPM or pricing structure for certain categories of health care services (typically high-volume, high-cost, or areas where specialty expertise can reduce costs for that segment, such as behavioral, sub-acute, lab, podiatry, chiropractic, X-ray, or transplants), not subject to discretionary utilization, and not included within the capitation rate; may also be created when a provider cannot or will not provide some segment of care, or is unavailable during periods of time when care may still be needed; geographically dispersed networks of specialists can form groups to attract carve outs; normally a carve out is warranted because there is special expertise and improved cost-effectiveness in a segment of care, versus lumping the segment in with an overall pricing

case management—*see CM*

case manager—a nurse, doctor, or social worker who works with patients, providers, and insurers to coordinate all services deemed necessary to provide the patient with a plan of medically necessary and appropriate care; *see also chronic disease center, and postdischarge case management*

case mix—a manner of describing the tendency of a group of covered lives to utilize services, in terms of the frequency and intensity of hospital admissions or services reflecting different needs and uses of hospital resources; case mix can be measured based on patients' diagnoses or the severity of their illnesses, the utilization of services, and the characteristics of a hospital; case mix influences ALOS, cost, and scope of services provided by a hospital

case rate—a reimbursement model used by hospitals to establish a flat rate per admission; the hospital sets rates based on an assumed average length of stay per admission, and the HMO is charged this rate for each member admitted; may have unique rates set or grouped by diagnosis type, or categories of medical/surgical, OB, critical care, or cardiac; other elements may include sliding scale volume, ALOS by type, volume of ancillary per patient, or contribution margin; *see also bundled case rate*

catastrophic insurance—protects the insured against all or a percentage of loss that is not covered by other insurance or prepayment plan or that is incurred under specified circumstances, or insurance in excess of specified amounts or other dollar or benefit limits

catchment area—the geographic area from which a plan draws its patients; under CHAMPUS, a zip code–specific area which normally conforms to a 40-mile radius circle surrounding a military treatment facility (MTF) that has financial responsibility for patients within the area; defines the population that may seek care from the MTF

categorically needy—aged, blind, or disabled persons or families and children under established financial thresholds of eligibility for "aid to families with dependent children (AFDC)," supplemental security income, or an optional state supplement

category-based pricing—a hospital reimbursement arrangement that provides a fixed pricing within a grouping of case types or DRG; *see also global per diem, DRG-specific per-case pricing, and global per diem*

center of excellence—health care institutions that have been credentialed and through clinical expertise and capital equipment improvements have proven to be able to provide a major resource intensive procedure in a more effective and efficient manner than made possible anywhere else within a defined region, such as for organ or bone marrow transplant, open heart surgery, high risk OB, or neonatal intensive care; such centers of excellence are listed in the *Federal Register*

certificate number—the number that identifies the person who is insured

certificate of authority—*see COA*

certificate of coverage—*see COC*

certificate of insurance—document delivered to an individual that summarizes the benefits and principal provisions of a group insurance contract

certificate of need—*see CON*

Certificate of Public Advantage law—*see COPA law*

certification—credentials; the statement that establishes that a person meets certain professional standards, issued by a board or association; the official authorization for use of services

CFR-42—code of federal regulations-42; the Public Health regulatory document that outlines procedures and requirements for federally qualified HMOs and CMPs, under HCFA and the Department of Health and Human Services

CHAMPUS—Civilian Health and Medical Program of the Uniformed Services; a federal program providing supplementary civilian-sector hospital and medical services beyond that which is available in military treatment facilities to military dependents, retirees and their dependents, and certain others; since the formation of this "standard" CHAMPUS program, added TRICARE contracts have been established with insurers who agree to provide managed care for beneficiaries within 1 of 12 regions in the United States; "standard" CHAMPUS is basically an indemnity-style insurance coverage—also called TRICARE Standard; *see also TRICARE, and wraparound plan*

CHAMPUS maximum allowable charge—*see CMAC*

channeling—the influence and practice by a patient broker, plan, provider, medical group, or physician to direct patients or workload away from one source to another; may be either the act of channeling to a different plan, provider, or hospital; *see also patient broker, physician channeling, physician channeling incentive, and specialist channeling*

channeling incentive—*see physician channeling incentive*

CHAP—Community Health Accreditation Program; originally the National League for Nursing's review function before its separate formation to serve as an accreditation authority for home care services; reviews customer satisfaction, clinical services, strategic management, and finances; *see also Joint Commission*

character-based terminal—the older type of computer terminal and system that supports only alphabetical or numeric characters, without the visual displays and "mouse"-driven bit-map software that most systems now utilize; the opposite of graphical user interface (GUI)

CHC—Community Health Center; providers of care for the needy at the community level as a safety net to other systems that do not provide services, either as federally qualified community centers that are guaranteed federal cost-based payment, or without this assistance; a growing number of CHCs are adding managed care features to their service, either independently or with the help of health plans; provide care, transportation, and translation services for uninsured, as well as commercial, Medicaid, and Medicare managed care patients; served by the trade association, the National Association of Community Health Centers; *see also FQHC*

chemical dependency services—treatment supplies and services in support of patients who are addicted to the classification of various chemicals, drugs, or alcohol, as listed by inclusion by the Department of Health and Human Services; *see also mental health carve out*

cherry picking—efforts by an insurer to gain favorable selection; state and federal governments are attempting to level the playing field against cherry picking through guaranteed issue, guaranteed renewal, and portability; *see also favorable selection, guaranteed issue, guaranteed renewal, and portability*

CHIN—community health information network; an electronic network to share medical information within a community of care entities, in a way that connects hospitals, clinics, rehab facilities, pharmacies, insurers, physicians, employers, and others having a need for the information; also called health information networks (HINs), regional health information networks (RHINs), enterprise information networks (EINs), and community health management information systems (CHMISs)

CHN—community health care network; *see CHIN*

chronic care capitation—involves payment to providers of chronic care, often includes specialist and facility care within the carve out; differs from a carve out capitated arrangement, in that the care is provided for a subset of patients who are known to be in need of chronic care, versus an entire population; suitable for HIV, chronic cardiac conditions, diabetes, severe asthma, but not for other chronic diseases that can be managed by a PCP; includes the responsibility for all health care needs for the chronic patient; *see also chronic care carve out*

chronic care carve out—involves a PMPM capitated payment to providers of chronic care, for all chronic health care needs of a given population; *see also chronic care capitation*

chronic disease center—a central location for a provider or a plan, which functions as a case manager for the aggressive management of chronic and high-risk patients, through the use of telephone contact and coordination of medical services requirements to ensure patients get care before their condition becomes aggravated, thereby reducing unnecessary medical costs, related to emergency room care, hospital admissions, physician visits, or other service charges; *see also CM*

churning—the method of patient care that emphasizes high productivity within a fee-for-service environment, in an attempt to increase provider revenue, either by seeing a patient more often than is medically necessary, or by creating unnecessary specialty referrals to colleagues

cigarette-related legislation—*see Measure 44*

CISN—Community Integrated Service Network; a recent effort in Minnesota that expands the community nonprofit, voluntary network concept of Integrated Service Networks (ISNs) to create licensed entities that combine insurance requirements with health care delivery (and PSN type structures) and allow greater competition between providers and insurers while discouraging overconsolidation by limiting enrollment to 50,000 per CISN; 10 CISNs are predicted in 12 months with various offerings for small groups and individuals, HMO, PPO, and POS formats; *see also CHIN, and PSN*

claim—the bill to a patient from the provider for medical services that were provided, from which processing for payment to the provider or patient is made; a demand to the insurers by or on behalf of an insured person for the payment of benefits under a policy; an act or omission that the insured reasonably believes will result in an express demand for damages to which this insurance applies

claims review—the validation process before payment, which consists of the medical appropriateness for care services rendered, and appropriate charge, accompanied by accurate and complete information

Clayton Act—(15 U.S.C., 13-19) establishes safeguards against health care entities crafting exclusivity or commodity sales that substantially lessen market competition; includes asset mergers, or joint ventures, consolidations, or acquisitions; goes beyond the Sherman Act by safeguarding what might happen, versus what actually has happened, to the market; *see also antitrust laws, and Sherman Act*

CLEAR—Consolidated Licensure for Entities Assuming Risk; an initiative begun by the NAIC in 1995 to establish a uniform set of requirements and definitions for various health plan entities; *see also NAIC, and unregulated provider entities*

clinic without walls—business operations (usually professional management services, group purchasing and support systems, centralized billing and accounting, uniform fee schedule, and the employment of all nonphysician staff), usually consisting of overhead items that have been consolidated among medical groups joining the network, are centralized while the delivery of care remains decentralized; *see also GPWW*

clinical algorithm—*see medical protocols*

clinical data information systems—automated systems that serve as a tool to inform clinicians about tests, procedures, and treatment, in an effort to increase efficiency, decrease managed health care utilization, without losing quality of care; clinical systems are becoming the fastest growth segment of the information systems industry, replacing financial and patient accounting emphasis of the past

clinical data repository—an automated data storage tool that acts as a file for retrievable patient data, which can be aggregated into reports or extracts to aid decision making, as an option to similar paper-based record functions; *see also data warehouse*

clinical mandate—benefits that health plans (other than under self-funded coverage) are required by state or federal law to provide and reimburse for policyholders and eligible dependents (begun under ERISA), such as in vitro fertilization, bone marrow transplants, a certain length of mental health or substance abuse treatment, or minimum maternity length of stay (even though the procedure may be considered experimental); *see also experimental, investigational, or unproven procedures, and maternity length of stay legislation*

clinical outlier—cases that cannot adequately be assigned to an appropriate DRG owing to unique combinations of diagnoses and surgeries, very rare conditions, or other unique clinical reasons; such cases are grouped together into clinical outlier DRGs; *see also cost outlier, and day outlier review*

clinical pathways—*see medical protocols*

clinical protocol—*see medical protocols*

closed access—a description that emphasizes the patient's restriction to an approved panel of providers; a managed care plan in which enrollees must select a primary care physician from the plan's participating providers; the patient is required to see only the approved PCPs for care, or to obtain referrals to other health care providers within the plan; this type of restricted provider access may be found in either group or staff HMOs; *see also closed panel, and gatekeeper model*

closed panel—a term with multiple applications that emphasize restriction of contracting partners or patients; a physician who no longer accepts new patients into a panel; a managed care plan that contracts with physicians on an exclusive basis for services and does not allow those physicians to see patients from another managed care organization; examples include staff and group model HMOs, and can apply to a large private medical group that contracts with a single HMO; physicians must normally meet narrow criteria or grant concessions in order to join an insurer's closed panel

closed PHO—more mature and exclusive model than the open PHO, in that not all providers are allowed to join, but rather those that have expertise in managing utilization and are continually approved as meeting certain standards; similar governance to open PHO, but more attractive to payers because of demonstrated cost reductions; increased feedback to providers to personal and peer practice utilization; this model does not contain the more advanced incentives of equity sharing from venture profits; *see also MSO, and open PHO*

CM—case management; the discipline directed toward the efficient and medically appropriate use of health care services for enrolled members, including either medical or ancillary health care resources; designed to achieve the optimal patient outcome in the most cost-effective manner; *see also PCCM*

CMAC—CHAMPUS maximum allowable charge; since CHAMPUS is the payer for the health care services received by a military member's family dependents in the civilian provider community, it establishes the maximum reimbursement rate paid to providers that "accept assignment"; these charges are set for each CPT code and DRG, and are adjusted annually

CMM—cumulative member months; an aggregate number used to quantify any given period of plan coverage representing the sum of the months multiplied by the members enrolled for each month

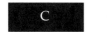

CMP—competitive medical plan; an approval given by HCFA (as a result of the 1982 TEFRA) to a prepaid health care entity that is willing to assume all financial risk and can meet all qualifications necessary to obtain a Medicare risk contract without having to obtain other added qualifications as an HMO; requirements for eligibility are somewhat less restrictive than an HMO; a legal entity organized under state law to deliver prepaid health care similar to an HMO; a CMP's package offering must include physician services, laboratory, X-ray, emergency, preventive, inpatient hospital, and out-of-area coverage; *see also HMO, and TEFRA*

CMS—care management system; a euphemism for a managed care system or even an IDN with support system infrastructure to manage practices, data, and clinical quality, with emphasis on adequate care with medically appropriate utilization rather than management and other organizational factors; an economically integrated health care provider network capable of delivering total health care for a defined population and assuming risk; seamless linkages between continuum of care options are highlighted within this discipline, together with multi-specialty patient attention and case management; *see also CM, and continuum of care*

COA—certificate of authority; issued by a state government to grant the license to an HMO to officially conduct operations

coalition—*see purchasing alliance*

COB—coordination of benefits; based on policy guidance within the National Association of Insurance Commissioners (NAIC) to prevent double payment for services when an enrollee has coverage from two or more sources; for example, a husband may have Blue Cross and Blue Shield through work, and the wife may have elected an HMO through her job—the COB agreement gives the order for what organization has primary responsibility for payment; used to ensure that the insured's benefits from all sources do not exceed 100% of allowable

COB recovery—when funds are recovered as a result of the elimination of unnecessary payment after coordination, in cases where COB did not initially preclude payment, contracts should contain language to show where this money goes (provider or HMO)

COBRA—Consolidated Omnibus Budget Reconciliation Act of 1985; a federal law requiring every hospital that participates in Medicare and has an emergency room to treat any patient in an emergency condition or active labor, whether or not covered by Medicare and regardless of ability to pay; COBRA also requires employers to provide continuation benefits to specified workers and families who have previously had benefits that have been terminated; *see also continuation*

COC—certificate of coverage; the basic document listing all health care benefits within the plan, as required by state law to reflect the contract as negotiated between employer and plan and shared with the employee

code of federal regulations-42—*see CFR-42*

coding—transferring narrative description of diseases, injuries, and medical procedures into numeric designations; *see also CPT*

coding creep—coding that is inappropriately elevated to generate a higher degree of reimbursement

coinsurance—a payment sharing arrangement between the insurance company or federal entity and the patient, which often includes the copayment concept of a specific amount per visit or for an established amount of supplies (such as $10 for a doctor visit or $5 for a 30-day prescription), or a stated percentage (such as the patient's 20% responsibility of payment); normally after a stated dollar amount of deductible is first met within the policy year deductible requirement, before which the patient pays all costs; additional costs above the usual, customary, and reasonable are paid by the member out of pocket; *see also copayment, and deductible*

COLA—cost of living adjustment; in 1974 Congress limited increases for Medicare Part B to the same percentage increase applied to Social Security cash benefits in the COLA, which is a reflection of general price inflation measured by the consumer price index; disability insurance has provisions to increase monthly benefits according to the COLA; *see also Medicare Part B premium share*

collections per thousand—a measure of the utilization of health care resources by a population at risk, derived by calculating the total collections for services divided by the number of covered lives within the group for a stated period of time, and then multiplying the result times one thousand

collective bargaining agreement—an agreement entered into between an employing entity and the bargaining representative of its employees, within the context of employee health benefits plans and HMOs

community care network—*see CHIN (community health integrated network); see also IDN*

Community Health Accreditation Program—*see CHAP*

Community Health Center—*see CHC*

Community Integrated Service Network—*see CISN*

community outreach—any activity by providers or insurers to bring education or medical services to the community, particularly in cases where the community lacks adequate understanding of, or access to primary and preventive health care services; can be provided through briefings, seminars, brochures, and or other written media that is appropriate for the linguistic and education level of the community; also effective when directed toward the building of trust, as an accurate and caring course of information, often delivered in partnership with other public and private agencies relating to cultural, employment, or political interests of the community; *see also geriatric outreach*

community rating—this method is required by HCFA for any federally qualified HMO to establish a premium level in a manner that does not take into account the actual claims experience of a group (as in experience rating), but predicts an insurance rate based on the average utilization of the entire community; many states have the same requirements for HMOs or even some indemnity plans; *see also ACR, adjusted community rate, and experience rating*

community rating by class—*see CRC*

community standard—often a primary determinant for what services should be offered within a community, as dictated by local expectations of accepted medical practice

comorbidity—the presence of a chronic condition or added complication other than the condition that requires medical treatment; within the context of DRGs, the comorbidity threshold causes an increase in ALOS by at least one day in 75% of admissions

competitive bidding—a method of price determination for health plan coverage that is based on gaining price information through a bidding process of competitors within a given geographical region; being considered by HCFA in a demonstration project that may yield wider application throughout the United States

competitive medical plan—*see CMP*

complementary benefits—benefits designed to work together with those of another program; Medicare recipients might enroll in Blue Shield programs that pay bills not covered by Medicare

complication—disease or condition arising during the course of, or as a result of, another disease, modifying medical care requirements; for DRGs, a condition that arises during the hospital stay that prolongs the length of stay by at least one day in approximately 75% of cases

component ware—application software that supports physician and patient information systems within a health "enterprise" by tying together multiple software objects that support departmental or functional processes; components may include laboratory, billing, referral trends, scheduling, or patient satisfaction functions

composite rate—the flat or standard rate that is charged to all enrollees of a health plan within a particular group, which constitutes a single charge for families or individuals

comprehensive health services—defined in Subpart A, 417.1 of the General Provisions portion of HCFA's federal regulation as a minimum of the following, which may be limited as to time and cost: physician services, outpatient services and inpatient hospital services, medically necessary emergency health services, and diagnostic laboratory and diagnostic and therapeutic radiology services

comprehensive medical expense insurance—form of health insurance that provides, in one policy, protection for both basic hospital expense and major medical expense coverage

computer-based patient record—*see electronic medical record*

Computer-Based Patient Record Institute—*see CPRI*

CON—certificate of need; a certificate of approval issued usually by a state health planning agency to health care facilities (in correlation with the National Health Planning and Resources Development Act of 1974) that propose to construct or modify a health care facility, incur a major capital expenditure, or offer a new or different health service; a key approach of cost containment used among the states; after a period of relaxed restrictions or free market direction, a Congressional repeal in 1986 and suspension of 11 state programs, attention has refocused in part on long-term care or raised spending thresholds, while other states still argue that the process is costly and fails to control costs; *see also COPN*

concurrent certification—*see admission certification*

concurrent review—a screening assessment of hospital admissions at the time they occur, performed by a professional managed care support staff during a patient's hospitalization, either by phone or through a representative's visit to the hospital location; this review is to make sure that utilization is appropriate; some health plans or providers require concurrent review for all admissions, while others require only a review on elective treatment and emergency admissions; *see also prospective review, and retrospective review*

conditionally renewable—insurance policy renewal provision that grants the insurer a limited right to refuse to renew a health insurance policy at the end of a premium payment period

confinement—language within a benefit contract that refers to an admission of a particular length that is uninterrupted; may be within an acute hospital, skilled nursing facility, or other inpatient facility

congregate living center—*see retirement residence*

Consolidated Licensure for Entities Assuming Risk—*see CLEAR*

Consolidated Omnibus Budget Reconciliation Act—*see COBRA*

consultative examiner—a physician who is paid a fee to examine and/or test a person for disability under either the SSDI or SSI program

consumer enrollment—*see Medicare open house recruitment and open enrollment period*

consumer retention—*see patient retention*

contact capitation—a relatively new method of full personal specialty capitation, which is an important variation on case rate; the capitation lump sum comes to the specialist only after first contact with a patient referred by a PCP; designed to include

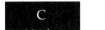

all care needed for the duration of the episode; should only be used with strong underutilization safeguards in place, due to the significant incentive; *see also individual specialist capitation, specialty capitation, and specialty department capitation*

continuation—extended benefits provided to enrolled members who have lost their employment or finalized a divorce that causes a loss of insurance benefits, allowed under specific insurance provisions for stated periods of extension; one of the provisions of COBRA, and a popular topic within the national health care debate for wider application to all employees

continued stay review—hospital or HMO UR activities certify the need for added length of stay through a continued stay review

continuing education—formal education pursued by a working professional and intended to improve or maintain professional competence

continuum of care—a spectrum of health care options, ranging from limited care needs through tertiary care, which has become the focus for an integrated delivery system to provide the appropriate expertise for the patient without providing a more expensive setting than necessary; an integrated delivery network can take full advantage of the continuum by ensuring good communication throughout the patient episode, and by using step-down, long-term care, rehab, sub-acute, or assisted living center features as soon as they provide an option over more costly hospitalization choices; *see also assisted living center, ICF, IDN, LTC, rehabilitation facility, and sub-acute care*

contract—a legally enforceable agreement between two parties of a health insurance policy

contract group—*see group*

contract mix—a breakout of a plan's enrollees by the number of dependents who are either single, married couple, or families of a certain size; used to determine average contract size

contract year—the beginning and ending period on the dates shown within a schedule of coverage, in which the dates are inclusive, normally at 12:01 standard time at the location of the plan

contracting alliance—*see purchasing alliance*

contractual allowance—a bookkeeping adjustment to reflect the difference between established charges for services rendered to insured persons and rates payable for those services under contracts with third-party payers (similar to a trade discount)

contribution coverage—*see contributory program*

contributory program or plan—an insurance payment structure in which the employer or local union pays part of the insurance premium, together with the employee, in order to make up the total premium amount required by the carrier; the employers make no commitment about specific benefits under this program

control plan—a Blue Shield plan that controls the administration of a health contract for an organization or employer within its geographic area, even though the employer has employees in other states

conversion factor—the dollar amount of one unit of service rendered that is used to convert various medical procedures into an established fee-schedule payment structure in which the conversion factor times the relative value unit creates the payment amounts; *see also RBRVS, RVS, and RVU*

conversion factor update—a yearly change to the official conversion factor stated above, established by Congress or a formula that measures actual expense growth from the past two years, and compares this growth to earlier predictions

conversion of enrollment—under HCFA guidelines, each HMO must offer individual enrollment to: each enrollee (and his or her enrolled dependents) leaving a group, and to each enrollee who would otherwise cease to be eligible for HMO enrollment because of his or her age, or the death or divorce of an enrollee

conversion, or conversion privilege—the privilege given to the covered person to change his/her coverage to a form of individual coverage without evidence of insurability; the condition for conversion can be made part of the master group contract; conversion is usually made when the patient leaves the group

cookbook medicine—the connotative description used by some to address the perceived excessive use of clinical protocols or other so-called best practice tools to aid provider decision making; *see also medical protocols, and triage algorithm*

cooling off period—a period that allows beneficiaries to change their mind regarding the selection of health care; specific draft language of a 120-day cooling off period was included in the 1995 House Ways and Means Subcommittee on Health regarding selection of MediSave, which could only be done during the "one chance" point of retirement, at which point a cooling off was offered to allow retirees to back out and optionally enroll in a managed care or FFS plan, or otherwise permanently forgo these options for MediSave; *see also MediSave*

cooperative care—term used when a patient is seen by a civilian physician or hospital for services that are cost-shared by CHAMPUS

coordinated care—a synonym or euphemism that has been used by the federal government to describe managed care

coordinated coverage—*see COB*

coordination of benefits—*see COB*

COPA law—Certificate of Public Advantage law; a state-level law, also called hospital cooperation act, which grants partners of approved joint ventures (and some mergers) a waiver from state and federal antitrust laws that would otherwise preclude the venture, assuming they meet a State Action Immunity test;

considered an easing of restriction on hospitals to aid their competition in the market, with 20 states approving COPAs since 1992; *see also state action immunity*

copayment—*see coinsurance*

COPN—certificate of public need; as an expanded definition used by some states in lieu of certificate of need, or CON, which highlights the need for public good to come out of additionally approved health services, whether they are added beds in a sub-acute facility, or a magnetic resonance imaging (MRI) machine; *see also CON*

cost allowance—charges recognized by a third-party payer that are incurred by health care providers in the usual course of providing health care services

cost-based reimbursement—the older payment methodology before either discounted FFS or any capitated structure; typically Blue Cross plans or government agencies, cost-based in the sense that the hospital or provider were paid their reasonable costs for delivered services as determined according to cost allocation and apportionment rules established by third-party payers; cost-based reimbursement is paid retrospectively, after all services have been rendered and a full accounting exercise has been accomplished for the hospital stay; the reimbursement will vary by hospital as determined by that hospital's cost structure and varying levels of reasonable costs; may be at either full cost, full cost plus percentage, allowable costs, or a fraction of costs

cost center—an accounting device that attributes all related costs to some "center" within a medical institution, such as the department of radiology, which might receive all direct costs attributable to that center, versus indirect or overhead costs that are spread among cost centers according to some formula

cost comparison data—data that show the comparative costs of providers offered by a growing number of state health authori-

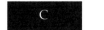

ties, local or regional authorities, or health plans to consumers; some providers include contract requirements for payers to send cost comparisons to enrolled members, knowing that their facility is a low-cost leader; *see also patient incentive, and physician channeling incentive*

cost compression—the generic description of a marketplace factor in which the amounts of revenue or premium are reduced (perhaps quite quickly) as managed care practices begin to occur; cost compression occurs due to pricing, utilization, and premiums

cost containment—a method or strategy to reduce health care costs

cost contract—used generically to describe the agreement between a plan and HCFA for managed care coverage of a membership population based on the reasonable costs of some of all Medicare covered benefits (as determined by the contract); typically a cost contract will involve monthly payments that may be adjusted to reflect actual data, and may include the use of AAPCC factors; now considered to be a less desirable reimbursement for the federal government, versus risk contracts, and currently proposed by the administration for repeal as of the year 2001

cost HMO—one of the three distinct types of managed care contracts with HCFA; cost HMOs are paid by Medicare and receive a predetermined monthly amount per beneficiary based on a total estimated budget, with adjustments at the end of the year for any variations from the budget; cost HMOs do not lock in Medicare enrollees into their networks, but are structured like point-of-service programs; Medicare will pay its share for non-plan providers (after the member's coinsurance and annual deductible just as in the traditional FFS system) but the cost HMO will not pay anything

cost of living adjustment—*see COLA*

cost outlier—a medical claim with an unusually high cost when compared with other discharges for the same DRG, within a statistical setting or established parameters; *see also clinical outlier*

cost per patient per day—the cost of running a health care facility divided by the number of inpatient days

cost sharing—a method of reimbursement for health care services that holds the patient responsible for a portion or percentage of the charge, with an attending strategy to serve as a means of reducing utilization; normally includes an annual deductible amount; *see coinsurance*

cost shifting—practice where a health care provider charges certain patients or third-party payers more for services in order to subsidize service provided below cost or free to the poor or uninsured, such as increasing "commercial pay patient" fees to cover indigent care losses

coverage decision—a health care payer's decision to either pay or reject payment for medical care to services, based on clinical information or the terms of the contract

covered expenses—those specific health care charges that an insurer will consider for payment under the terms of a health insurance policy; *see also covered services*

covered lives—refers to the quantity of persons who are enrolled within a particular health plan, or for coverage by a provider network; includes enrollees and their covered dependents

covered persons—*see covered lives*

covered services—a written health care benefit document that outlines the benefit package to be provided to either individual beneficiaries or a purchasing group or employer, with a corresponding sum for each service; services specified for beneficiaries by an insurer, HCFA, or equivalent state program for Medicaid entitlements, in a benefit plan or managed care contract; specific services and supplies for which the federal or commercial payer will provide reimbursement; these may consist of a combination of mandatory and optional services within each state

CPR—computer-based patient record; *see electronic medical record*

CPR—customary, prevailing, and reasonable charges; the Medicare methodology for paying physicians from 1965 until the January 1992 implementation of Medicare fee schedule policy; the lowest amount for either the billed amount, the customary charge, or the prevailing community charge was reimbursed by Medicare; superseded by the RBRVS Medicare fee schedule; *see also RBRVS*

CPRI—Computer-Based Patient Record Institute; a recommendation came from a study of the National Academy of Science's Institute of Medicine in 1991 to form this joint public–private sector effort, to promote and facilitate development, implementation, and dissemination of the computer-based patient record; located in Chicago

CPT—Current Procedural Terminology; unique sets of five-digit codes that apply to the medical service or procedure performed by physicians and other providers; the system of coding for physicians' services, established by the CPT Editorial Panel of the AMA, has become the industry coding standard for reporting

CPT-4—Current Procedural Terminology, 4th edition; *see also CPT*

CR—carrier replacement; occurs whenever one insurer replaces another insurer or multiple insurers for a particular group of covered lives; adding to a carrier's covered population is beneficial in the sense that a large group will call for lower levels of stop-loss coverage or other related costs because of the larger group experience and the spreading of risk among more patients

CRC—community rating by class; a form of community rating in which separate groups of enrollees can have different actuarial premium rates depending on the age, sex, marital status, and industry component of the group under review; still not equivalent to experience rating, in that there is no actual cost experience for the specific group of patients under review; *see also experience rating*

credentialing—the review process leading to the ultimate granting of medical privileges to a provider, by a hospital or insurer; a careful review of documents, medical license, relevant certificates, evidence of malpractice insurance (in cases where the insurance is needed or not provided by the supporting hospital or HMO by agreement), any history involving actual or alleged malpractice, and educational background of professional providers; may apply to seeking candidacy on care panels

credentialing function outsourcing—a growing number of companies serve as consultants to managed credentialing functions for a group practice, hospital, IDN, IPA, HMO, or other type of physician network; services include virtually all requirements for NCQA accreditation, such as ensuring the review of: license to practice, hospital privileges, Drug Enforcement Agency registration, sanctions by Medicare/Medicaid, malpractice claims history and insurance coverage, medical education/residency/boards, and application processing; they also may perform on-site reviews and establish necessary links with the NPDB and AMA; *see also NCQA, and NPDB*

credentialing negligence—the credentialing of a provider without adequate review of background, malpractice history, and licensure; may also apply to the selection of a utilization review organization with subsequent problems

credentials verification organization—*see credentialing function outsourcing*

critical care—health care provided to critically ill patients during a medical crisis, usually within a critical care area such as an intensive care unit or coronary care unit

critical pathways—*see medical protocols*

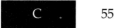

crossover claim—a bill for services rendered to a patient receiving benefits simultaneously from Medicare and Medicaid or other carriers, in which Medicare pays first and then determines the amounts of unmet Medicare deductible and coinsurance to be paid by Medicaid; *see also dual eligible*

Current Procedural Terminology—*see CPT*

custodial care—care that is not directed toward a cure or restoration to a previous state of health (as in acute care) but includes medical or nonmedical services provided to maintain a given level of health without skilled nursing care; *see also assisted living center, and continuum of care*

customary charge—the amount that a physician usually charges the majority of patients

customary, prevailing, and reasonable—*see CPR*

customer satisfaction—*see patient satisfaction*

cycle time—used to describe the turnaround time (TAT) from start to finish for a particular process, such as claims processing; *see also TAT*

daily service charge—*see per diem reimbursement*

data warehouse—*see clinical data repository*

database management system—*see DBMS*

date of plan insolvency—the later date of either of the following, provided both occur: the date on which a court of competent jurisdiction formally declared finds the plan to be insolvent, and the date on which the plan ceases all operations

date of service—*see DOS*

DAW—dispense as written; the instruction from a physician to a pharmacist to dispense a brand-name pharmaceutical rather than a generic substitution

day outlier review—a review of potential day outliers (short or unusually long ALOS) to determine the necessity of admission and the number of days before the day outlier threshold is reached as well as the number of days beyond the threshold; additional days are approved by the Peer Review Organization

days per thousand—same as bed days/1,000; a standard unit of measurement of use of health care services; refers to an annualized use of the hospital or other institutional care; the number of hospital days used in a year for each thousand covered lives; derived by first taking the number of bed days divided by member months, and then multiplying by each 1,000 members, also multiplied by the number of months under consideration

DBMS—database management system; a system that supports the rapid and flexible retrieval or analysis of medical data, by keeping the data file separated from other computer applications that may be used to collect or process the data

DC—dual choice; Congress enacted dual choice within Title 13 of the Public Health Service Act, so that employers of 25 or more persons with employees residing in an HMO's service area must pay minimum wage and offer their employees health benefits to which they contribute, and must give employees the option of joining an HMO, in addition to providing indemnity insurance coverage as a basic entitlement; the employer must give the HMO marketing opportunities at least equal to those given the current indemnity carrier (dual choice does not apply to CMPs); employers are not required to offer multiple HMOs of the same type unless the second HMO can prove that it has a unique service area

DCA—Deferred Compensation Administrator; a firm that offers an array of compensation planning, workers' compensation claims administration, retirement planning services, third-party administration, and self-insured plan services

DCA—Dependent Care Account; within the structure of employee flexible spending accounts that meet Internal Revenue Service criteria; employers maintain a separate account for family members, called Dependent Care Accounts or DCAs (separate from the account for the employees, called Health Care Accounts); *see also flexible spending account, and HCA*

DCG—diagnostic cost groups; a system of Medicare reimbursement for HMOs with risk contracts in which enrollees are classified into various DCGs on the basis of each beneficiary's prior 12-month hospitalization history

DCI—duplicate coverage inquiry; occurs when one insurance company makes a request to another insurance company to see if overlapping coverage exists on a subscriber, for purposes of coordination of benefits to make sure that unnecessary payments are not made

DDS—Disability Determination Services; a state Social Security division office that assesses a case for disability benefits

death spiral—refers to a sequential spiral of high premium rates and adverse selection that causes financial losses for an insurer, because underwriting losses rise faster than the premiums can recover; can also refer to an economic reference for medical practices that do not learn to modify provider behavior toward managed care efficiencies in time to remain competitive with the competition

deductible—the minimum threshold payment that must be made by the enrollee each year before the plan begins to make payments on a shared or total basis; the amount the Loss of Plan must sustain for each member in each contract year for each category of coverage before any benefits become payable under the agreement; if an enrollee has a $100 annual deductible, no payment assistance comes from the plan until at least a total of $101 in eligible claims are processed within the calendar or contract year; plans will typically reduce the deductible if they wish to create an added incentive for patients to enroll, or they use reduced deductibles as the initial means to get reluctant patients to try some form of managed care

deductible carryover credit—for plans that include a carryover credit, the acceptable health care charges for services during the last three months of a calendar year may be used as a credit toward the next year's deductible

deemed status—initially, the "deemed status" was a way to recognize a hospital or other health care organization as being approved, in the sense that allowed Medicare or Medicaid reimbursement by virtue of an accreditation certification, as practiced by the Joint Commission since 1965; although there was not comparable mandate for HMOs despite pioneer programs by the Joint Commission and NCQA, the current draft Dec 95 Administration proposal of Medicare revisions contains quality assurance provisions, as accredited by private entities meeting the Secretary's standards; *see also Joint Commission, NCQA, and Quality Assurance*

DEERS—Defense Enrollment Eligibility Reporting System (DEERS), a Department of Defense program that provides, among other services, an electronic database to verify beneficiary eligibility; the system that is used to determine eligibility (in addition to the military identification card) for TRICARE or traditional military treatment facility care

Deferred Compensation Administrator—*see DCA*

defined contribution coverage—*see contributory program or plan*

delete—the removal of an enrollee from a health care plan, according to stated procedures or time limitations within the contract

delinquent claim—insurance claim submitted to an insurance company, for which payment is overdue; claim not submitted on time to a carrier

demand management—a discipline that is directed toward assisting the consumer to know how to make an appropriate use of medical services; includes many strategies designed to ensure patient care quality while reducing traditional demand upon a primary care physician, such as: workplace health promotion or wellness programs, lifestyle management or behavioral change to avoid or reduce health risks, self-management of minor acute conditions through awareness of alternate treatment guidebooks, or self help to assist in group or individual management of chronic conditions; decision support systems to support demand management include: telephone-based hotlines, trained nurse counselors, and information and psychosocial support for informed choice

demonstration projects—these tests of prospectively determined managed care arrangements have been pursued under sections of the Social Security Amendments for Medicare enrollees, and also enacted by Congress for analysis through Department of Defense efforts; examples include Medicare Choice demonstration, the Tidewater, Virginia CHAMPUS demonstration for mental health, and the CHAMPUS Reform Initiative (CRI); *see also Medicare+Choice*

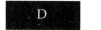

denial and reconsideration—if HCFA denies an application for qualification, it gives the entity written notice of the denial and an opportunity to request reconsideration, if submitted in writing within 60 days following denial with content to address denial issues

denied claim—insurance claim submitted to an insurance company in which payment has been rejected due to either a technical error or the failure of the care rendered to quality for coverage under the plan; ERISA claims denials require a reason, with specific reference of provisions for denial, added information needed for coverage and why information is needed, and instructions for appeal; *see also ERISA*

dental care—a common additional benefit offered by HMOs; *see additional benefits to Medicare risk*

dental carve out—the specific reference to dental care that is a carve out segment of the PMPM or contract pricing, which may require that oral surgeons be participating providers in the case that oral surgery is included

department capitation—*see specialty department capitation*

Department of Health and Human Services—*see HHS*

dependent—an enrolled health plan member who has coverage tied to that of the sponsor; may be a spouse or an unmarried child, or a stepchild or legally adopted child of either the employee or the employee's spouse, whose primary domicile is with the employee, except for other arrangements as approved by the plan; often dependent children status is also delineated by those under the age of 18, or children attending college full-time under a specified age

Dependent Care Account—*see DCA*

deselection of providers—*see exclusivity*

desk review—the first step of HCFA's procedures to federally qualify an HMO or CMP; following the completeness screen of the application, the HCFA review specialists will prepare a written report of findings, with a copy mailed to the applicant for subsequent discussions on-site; review reports may include requests for additional documentation or requested interviews to be conducted while on-site

determination of qualification or eligibility—the fourth and final step of HCFA's procedures to federally qualify an HMO or CMP, involving a decision by the Director of the Office of Qualification in consultation with the Director of the Office of Compliance and the Deputy Director of the Office of Prepaid Health Care; determination decisions may include "determination of qualifiability or eligibility," "60-day notice of intent to deny," or "denial"

DFFS—discounted fee-for-service; a payment method that is calculated as a certain percentage of discount from fee-for-service charges; among the least risky contracting approaches, second only to billed charges; may include a sliding scale tied to volume, with varying discounts by product line; similar to full FFS except that the HMO agrees to pay billed hospital charges, or outpatient services, minus a fixed percentage, which is based on the efficiencies of guaranteed payments, usage protocols used by the HMO; *see also FFS, and global capitation*

diagnosis protocols—a subset of medical protocols that deals with the detection of disease; protocols outline a recommended set of examinations and tests, with corresponding index of diagnosis alternatives that are likely to be present, based upon the results; *see also medical protocols, prevention protocols, and treatment protocols*

diagnostic category—*see medical diagnostic category*

diagnostic cost group—*see DCG*

diagnostic creep—*see coding creep*

direct access care systems or contracting—*see direct contracting*

direct capitation—*see full personal capitation*

direct care—a term used within the Department of Defense to describe care provided within the military treatment facility

direct contract model—*see direct contracting*

direct contracting—one of multiple relationships between payers and providers, or purchasers and providers, that omits an intermediate party that is present in most other contracts of its type; first example—a health plan that contracts directly with private practice physicians, or provider groups in the community, rather than through an intermediary such as an IPA or a medical group; common among open panels; second example—the practice of providing care under the direct agreement between employers or business coalitions and providers, also called direct access system, with no HMO or PPO intermediary; normally hospitals offer price discounts and employers agree to limit the number of providers while creating incentives for employees to use in-network providers; some employers offer vouchers or fixed health care funds to employees, then allow employees to select the system; *see also cafeteria plan, ODS, and PSN*

direct costs—costs that are entirely attributed to a service, such as the professional and equipment costs charged to obstetrics

direct mail—a marketing technique that may be used by physicians, providers, and insurers to inform patients about the benefits of managed care, to provide education about various types of coverage or products, and to influence the patient's decision in a way that causes the use of the marketer's product, services, or causes some other type of health care consumption; *see also personal letter*

direct service contract—a contract for the provision of basic or supplemental health services or both between an HMO and either a health professional (other than a member of the staff of the HMO) or an entity other than a medical group or an IPA

dirty claims—those medical claims that contain errors that preclude automated processing before problems are resolved or the claim is rejected; also called "other" or "dingy" claims

disability—physical or mental condition that makes an insured person incapable of performing one or more occupational duties either temporarily, long-term, or totally

disability income insurance—form of health insurance that provides periodic payments when an insured person is unable to work as a result of illness or injury

disabled—any physical or mental condition that renders an insured person unable to do work for which he or she is qualified and educated; eligibility for Medicare disability begins at the two-year point for disabled under 65 entitled under either the Social Security Act or the railroad retirement system; *see also total disability*

discharge planning—the activity that occurs early in the admission process to evaluate the patient's medical needs in order to reduce LOS and to arrange for appropriate care after discharge from an inpatient setting, to include selection of LTC, subacute, home health, transportation, and other support service requirements; before specific emphasis was recently placed on discharge planning, patients often were ready for discharge from an acute hospital setting but still required care from a lower point along the continuum—but because plans had not been made in advance and no facility was available on short notice, patients were forced to remain in the hospital at a higher cost than would have been necessary within an alternate setting; *see also continuum of care, and LOS*

discharge planning–placement coordinator—a staff member of a provider or health plan, responsible for discharge planning functions, which can begin upon the patient's acute hospitalization; often staffed by a nurse, social worker, or other staff member with special training or expertise; *see also discharge planning*

discharge summary—an admission summary prepared at the time of the patient's discharge from the hospital

discount from full charges—*see DFFS*

discounted fee-for-service charges—*see DFFS*

disease management measures—indicators of a health plan's success in treating the entirety of a disease across the continuum of care—related to the family of outcome measures that treat the disease as opposed to managing health; may include measures for major diagnostic categories (hypertension, diabetes, heart disease), primary care (patient satisfaction with service, utilization of preventive services, illness episodes per 1,000), specialty care (diagnostic or therapeutic guidance compliance, visits per 1,000, diagnosis-specific health status scores), acute care episodes (ALOS per major DRG categories, surgeries per 1,000, readmission rates) or rehab and recovery (patient compliance, DRG-specific health status scored)

disenrollment—the process of terminating coverage; normally, voluntary disenrollment is not allowed until the patient has remained within the plan for at least 6–12 months; a patient can be involuntarily disenrolled because of a change in employment; Medicare seniors may disenroll at the beginning of any given month, assuming notice is given by a certain preceding deadline during the previous month

dismemberment—the accidental loss of limb or sight

disproportionate share hospital—*see DSH*

DME—durable medical equipment; equipment that can endure repeated use, without being subject to disposal after one-time use (such as insulin pumps, wheelchairs, home hospital beds, walkers, glaucometers, motor-driven wheelchairs, or oxygen equipment); generally DME is not useful or needed by a person in the absence of illness or injury

doctors referral line—*see physician referral service*

documentation—chronological detailed record of pertinent facts and observations about a patient's health as seen in chart notes and medical reports

DoD/HCFA tests for military BRAC sites—for 12 locations in the states of AZ, CA, FL, IN, MA, PA, and TX, the Department of Defense and HCFA are testing an alternate program for retirees over 65 and their dependents who have been affected by base realignment and closure (BRAC); although retirees 65 and older lose CHAMPUS eligibility when they become eligible for Medicare, they are still seen in military treatment facilities (MTFs) on a space-available basis; this program offers members enrollment in locally available Medicare HMOs as a means to substitute their loss of the MTF, providing contact information through DEERS regarding Medicare enrollment and coverage details; chronic drugs are also offered through the TRICARE contractor for two years after base closure; *see also CHAMPUS, DEERS, HCFA, and MTF*

dollar rate—one of two factors used to calculate the payment under the DRG prospective payment system

donation rules—current legislative proposals for Medicaid reform involving block grants to the state, either with the presence or elimination of donation rules, which prohibit the practice of state-level donations from Medicaid providers as a strategy to increase federal matching; *see also Medicaid state matching rate*

DOS—date of service; the day of health care service to an enrolled beneficiary

double indemnity—the feature in some disability policies that requires the payment of twice the policy's normal benefit, or face amount, in case of loss resulting from specified causes or conditions

downstream costs—typically used to describe all costs that are directly or indirectly incurred by a PCP, and normally involve

notions about how to reduce or control utilization of those costs as a solution for better efficiency in managing care for populations; include inpatient services, referrals to specialists, diagnostic procedures, mental health, pharmacy, and all other costs that occur subordinate to the PCP; *see also full personal capitation, PCP, and PCR*

DPR—drug price review; a weekly update of the average wholesale price of drugs, which is provided through the American Druggist Blue Book; the review process leads to the creation of price ceilings, in the maximum allowable price list; *see also AWP, and MAC list*

dread disease policy—health coverage that may involve a rider or supplement to provide benefits for specific disease categories as listed

DRG—diagnosis or diagnostic-related groups; a Yale University-derived system of classification for 383 inpatient hospital services based on principal diagnosis, secondary diagnosis, surgical procedures, age, sex, and presence of complications; this system is used as a financing mechanism to reimburse hospital and selected other providers for services rendered; used to describe patient mix in hospitals and to determine hospital reimbursement policy

DRG 468-470—DRGs of 468, 469, 470, and 477 have shown particular value for workload analysis, so they are reviewed here: 468—extensive operating room (OR) procedures unrelated to the principal diagnosis; 469—principal diagnosis invalid or unmatched as discharge diagnosis; 470—errors in the record make the diagnosis ungroupable; and 477—nonextensive OR procedure unrelated to principal diagnosis

DRG creep—*see coding creep*

DRG rate—a fixed dollar amount based on an average of all patients in a specific DRG in the base year adjusted for inflation, economic factors, and bad debts; *see also DRG*

DRG risk pool—*see hospital DRG risk pool*

DRG-specific per-case pricing—a type of fixed-per-case pricing system used by hospitals to charge a fixed amount for a specific DRG; the basic structure used by Medicare; DRG-specific pricing allows limitation of risk by identifying extraordinary LOS cases separately; *see also category-based pricing, and global fee*

DRG weight—an index number assigned to each DRG to reflect the relative cost for all hospitals for treating cases within that DRG

drug formulary—*see formulary*

drug maintenance list—*see additional drug benefit list*

drug price review—*see DPR*

drug utilization review—*see DUR*

DSH—disproportionate share hospital; the share of a hospital's expenses that is directed toward the care of the indigent, according to the definition of U.S. Code, Title 42, Chapter 7, subchapter XIX, "Grants to States for Medical Assistance Programs"; hospitals that serve a disproportionate number of low income patients with special needs

dual choice—*see DC*

dual eligible—used to describe a beneficiary who is eligible for Medicare and Medicaid, and under the proposed MediGrant policy would be eligible for Medicare and MediGrant within a set aside program funding; used within the Department of Defense to describe a beneficiary who has dual health care entitlement as both a military retiree and a Medicare eligible; *see also set aside*

dual option—*see dual choice; see also triple option*

due diligence—a review or investigation by a prospective party to a contract, such as a hospital evaluating a contract with a managed care organization or a physician practice to be acquired, to ensure financial stability, proper legal structure to enter into a contract, reputation, adequate supplier–provider relationships, and acceptable reimbursement or equity sharing strategy for the resulting contract

duplicate coverage inquiry—*see DCI*

duplication of benefits or coverage—partially or totally duplicate coverage under two or more plans for the same potential loss, usually the result of contracts with different service organizations, insurance companies, or prepayment plans

DUR—drug utilization review; a quantitative review to establish the medical appropriateness of providers giving medications to patients for particular medical conditions, performed by peers with feedback and education given to the providers, as appropriate

durable medical equipment—*see DME*

DXNNH—diagnosis not normally hospitalized

E codes—a classification of ICD-9-CM coding for external causes of injury rather than disease; E codes are also used in coding adverse reactions to medications

E of I—*see EOI*

ear examinations—a common additional benefit to members enrolled in HMO plans; *see additional benefits to Medicare risk*

Early and Periodic Screening, Diagnosis, and Treatment—*see EPSDT*

earned premium—portion of a premium for which protection of the policy has already been provided by the insurer

EBITDA—earnings before interest, taxes, depreciation, and amortization; many merger and acquisition deals involving nonprofit hospitals as the acquired entity use this method to value the hospital's earnings before these factors are taken into consideration

EDI—electronic data interchange; the electronic transfer of claims data or other information between two or more health care organizations; payers and providers are making an increased use of EDI

effective date—the date a contract becomes enforced; may apply to the relationship between the plan and the employer, or between the plan and the enrollee; *see also eligibility date*

effectiveness—the overall health benefit to a patient that is provided by a medical care or service within a community practice setting

efficacy—the overall health benefit reached under ideal conditions for selected patients

EGHP—Employer Group Health Plan; a private, employment-originated health plan covering an individual who also has Medicare coverage due to being age 65 or over, in which Medicare is the secondary payer

electronic claim—insurance claim submitted to the carrier by a central processing unit, tape diskette, direct data entry, direct wire, dial-in telephone, digital fax, or personal computer download or upload; *see also EDI*

electronic data interchange—*see EDI*

electronic medical record—*see EMR*

eligibility date—the day on which an enrollee is first entitled to health care benefits according to a contract

eligibility list—a list that shows the eligible enrolled members for health care services and supplies, including their effective date; *see also effective date*

eligibility period—time following the eligibility date (usually 31 days) during which a member of an insured group may apply for insurance without evidence of insurability

eligible dependent—*see dependent*

eligible employee—health plan contracts outline requirements for an employee to meet eligibility requirement in the health plan, which are based on factors such as full-time or part-time employment as stipulated in the contract

eligible expenses—the usual, customary, and reasonable charges or established rates for health care or supplies covered or allowed under a health plan; do not include copayments to any source, or amounts paid by the member under the membership service agreement

eligible hospital services—medically necessary hospital services that are provided to a member in a hospital on a day for which

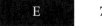

there is a room and board charge, prescribed by a licensed physician, and rendered according to the membership service agreement; include referral services, but are not deemed to include physicians' or surgeons' charges unless specifically included in an endorsement

emergency—life endangering bodily injury or sudden and unexpected illness that requires a member to seek immediate medical attention under circumstances that effectively preclude seeking care through a plan physician or a plan medical center; immediate care needed to preserve life, loss of limb, eyesight, bodily tissue, or to preclude unnecessary pain and suffering; *see also emergency services*

emergency services—an important definition that determines whether care will be reimbursed; may involve care within a plan, as defined by the above definition for "emergency"; or may address those services that are essentially out-of-area emergencies; HCFA defines as covered inpatient or outpatient services that are furnished by an appropriate source other than the HMO or CMP for care needed immediately because of injury or sudden illness, when such care cannot be delayed for the time required to reach the HMO or CMP provider or authorized alternative without risk of permanent damage to the patient's health, and when transfer to an HMO or CMP source is also precluded because of risk or unreasonable distance, given the nature of the medical condition; many believe that a standard definition should be developed at the state or federal level; *see also out-of-area emergency, and prudent layperson*

emergency symptoms—the basis for proposed reimbursement criteria for emergency patient claims to managed care organizations, versus the emergency diagnosis, but not yet enacted in any state; *see also prudent layperson*

emergi-center—*see free-standing emergency medical service center*

employee—any individual employed by an employer or public entity on a full-time or part-time basis; *see also eligible employee*

employee contribution—the portion of the health care premium that is the responsibility of the employee, according to contract or terms of employment

Employee Retirement Income Security Act—*see ERISA*

employee welfare plan—*see ERISA plan*

employer—a fairly wide definition, patterned after the entities listed within the 1938 Fair Labor Standards Act and Internal Revenue Code, including nonappropriated fund entities and excluding the governments of the United States, District of Columbia, and the territories and possessions of the United States, the 50 states and their political subdivisions, the U.S. Postal Service and Postal Rate Commission, and church-related entities

employer coalition—*see purchasing alliance*

employer contribution—the portion of the health care premium that is the responsibility of the employer; the employer contribution may vary based on tenure or family status, or other factors that may be stipulated by the employer

Employer Group Health Plan—*see EGHP*

employer health fair—*see health fair*

employer mandate—essentially, the mandate for an employer to provide a dual choice option for employees to have access to health care; *see also dual choice*

employer–provider risk pool—*see provider–employer risk pool*

employing entity—either an employer or public entity; *see also employer, and public entity*

EMR—electronic medical record; an automated, on-line medical record that is available to any number of providers, ancillary service departments, pharmacies, and others involved in patient treatment or care; as a result of computer technology that stores, processes, and retrieves patient clinical and demographic information upon request of the user; pioneered at locations like Duke University Hospital for eliminating problems of redundancy or illegibility, reducing human error, streamlining data entry, and centralizing the management of a patient record

encounter—a health care visit of any type that warrants payment of services by an enrollee to a provider of care or services

encounter outcomes measures—measures of the results of specific clinical encounters (e.g., inpatient or outpatient surgical procedures, outpatient diagnostic tests, emergency department visits)

encounter per member per year—the annual number of encounters for an enrollee, as an average of all enrollees in the plan

encounter record—another word for a claim; also refers to a patient visit information record

end-stage renal disease—*see ESRD*

enrollee—a covered member of a health care contract who is eligible to receive contract services; *see also insured*

enrollee health status measures—indicators of a health plan's ability to maintain the health of its enrollee population

enrolling unit—the unit level of enrollment may be either at an individual employer or other group entity level, involving the signing of a contract for health care coverage

enrollment—the number of patients who have contracted with a carrier; the process or activity of actually recruiting and signing up individuals and groups for membership in a plan; a description of the number of covered lives in a plan

enrollment broker—*see patient broker*

enrollment card—a card-type document that serves as notice that an employee wishes to participate in an employer group insurance plan

enrollment health fair—*see health fair*

enrollment lock-in period—the minimum period of time enrollees must maintain enrollment in a plan, after the initial date of enrollment, before they are eligible to disenroll; lock-in periods vary by plan, ranging from no-lock in, to a month, half year, or year or more

enrollment period—*see federal open enrollment, group enrollment period, and open enrollment period*

enrollment retention—*see patient retention*

EOB—explanation of benefits; the description of provided services that is sent to enrolled members of a plan in an attempt to clarify the coverage entitlements and charges; the traditional health care payment system under which physicians and other providers receive a payment that does not exceed their billed charge for each unit of service provided; an EOB consists of a statement that tells what and why various services were or weren't covered

EOI—evidence of insurability; proof presented through written statements (i.e., an application form) and/or a medical examination that an individual is eligible for a certain type of insurance coverage, in terms of not having pre-existing conditions that would likely cause immediate claims against the carrier; this form is required for eligibles who do not enroll during the open enrollment period or who apply for excess amounts of group life insurance; also called evidence of good health

episode—includes all health care treatment and expenditures surrounding an admission as an inpatient, partial hospitalization, or outpatient treatment; the analysis of episode costs is generally conducted by selecting some reasonable but arbitrary period of time surrounding the event, and relating all costs to that episode, such as treatment between admission and discharge, or any care received within 14 days from the days of admission

EPO—exclusive provider organization; a term derived from the phrase preferred provider organization (PPO) and similar in

construction within states that allow EPOs; however, although a patient may go outside the network for care, the patient must remain in the network to receive benefits (out of network care results in payment by the patient); a plan regulated under state insurance statute that only provides coverage for contracted providers and does not extend to nonpreferred provider services

EPSDT—Early and Periodic Screening, Diagnosis, and Treatment; a screening and diagnostic program with the specific focus toward recipients under 21 years of age, which reviews any physical or mental problems and the associated medical requirements to address these problems

ERISA—Employee Retirement Income Security Act; this 1974 federal law mandates reporting and disclosure requirements for group life and health plans, with relevant guidance on the sponsorship, administration, minimum record retention period, servicing of plans, some claims processing, appeals regulations, and minimum mandatory clinical benefits; ERISA removes self-insured health plans from the various state legislation regarding health insurance; *see also clinical mandate*

ERISA plan—within the context of insurance benefits for employees (29 U.S.C., 1002(1)), ERISA plans provide for the variety of medical, surgical, hospitalization, disability, death, unemployment, and other benefits

ESRD—end-stage renal disease; patients determined to have ESRD are not eligible to enroll in an HMO or CMP except as specified in section 417.434 of CFR-42 concerning reenrollment, unless they were an HMO enrollee at the time they became eligible for Medicare

Ethics in Patient Referral Act—*see Stark I*

evidence of coverage—a description of the benefits within the plan; covered by state laws and represents the coverage provided under the contract issued to the employer, the evidence is provided to the employee; also called certificate of coverage

evidence of insurability—*see EOI*

excluded hospitals—hospitals excluded from the prospective payment system that will continue to receive payments from Medicare on the basis of reasonable cost subject to the target rate of increase limits

exclusion—the practice of keeping an entity out of a network for the purpose of eliminating poor health care; may be conducted by an insurer with regard to hospitals, or by a PHO, or PPO with regard to individual physicians or group practices; *see also exclusivity*

exclusion coverage—health care benefit coordination or integration provided by Medicare and an employer; Medicare payments are subtracted from actual claims and the employer-sponsored plan's benefits are applied to the balance

exclusion safeguards—some providers take measures to prevent exclusion from a health plan, by voicing appeals or concerns to influential community leaders, members of their own governance board, leaders of local corporations, or directly to the employees or patients; assuming sufficient and credible pressure is created, the provider may avoid exclusion from the network

exclusions—health care conditions specified in the contract or employee benefit plan for which the plan will not provide payment

exclusive provider organization—*see EPO*

exclusivity—occurs in situations where a hospital or provider convinces an HMO to limit the network (or when an insurer purposefully limits a network), so that they are the only provider, or one of an extremely small number of providers; the hospitals normally concede discounts in exchange for exclusivity in hopes of increased volume in return; there appears to be less desire by payers to seek exclusive deals, especially in early market development; *see also AWP laws, sliding price scale, and two-way exclusives*

expansion of services—the addition of any health service not previously provided by or through the HMO that requires an increase in the facilities, equipment, or health professionals of the HMO; or the improvement or upgrading of existing facilities or equipment, or an increase in the number of categories of health professionals of the HMO so that the HMO could provide directly services that it previously provided through contract or referral or which it couldn't previously provide with its existing facilities or equipment; *see also significant expansion*

expected claims—essentially the best-guess projection of the cost of health care and services for an individual enrollee or a group of members; based on the same type of actuarial projections as experience rating data, and also within the context of the medical loss ratio or cost of actual care (versus administrative, claims processing, and overhead) over a particular contract duration; *see also experience rating*

experience—*see MLR*

experience rating—the methodology for establishing a future premium level that is derived from previous data for the actual costs of care and services for a group of enrollees, versus the alternative of the community rating system mandated by HCFA for federally qualified HMOs; *see also community rating*

experimental, investigational, or unproven procedures—experimental procedures are specifically excluded from most health plan coverage, since there is little or speculative evidence that these treatments are effective, or proven in the treatment of the condition; HMOs look to entities such as the AMA, FDA, DHHS, National Institutes of Health, or the Council of Medical Specialty Societies to confirm the ultimate value of health care procedures, services, medical supplies and equipment, or drug interventions

experimental treatment legislation—legislation is now being drafted that attempts to reach some common ground between the patient's need for experimental treatment that has a reasonable chance of success, and the managed care organization's need to avoid costly, nonessential treatment

explanation of benefits—*see EOB*

extended care facility—a facility that is licensed by applicable state or local law to offer room and board, skilled nursing by a full-time registered graduate nurse (RN), intermediate care, or a combination of levels on a 24-hour basis; may be an institution that is owned, operated by, or affiliated with a hospital, a separate and distinct part of a hospital, any other institution or part of an institution meeting the requirements established for approved operation under Medicare; commonly an ex-tended care facility does not include a clinic, a rest home, a home for the aged, a place for treatment of alcoholism or drug abuse, or a place for custodial care; *see also continuum of care*

extension of benefits—before the COBRA regulations (which include certain protection for employees and their families that were impacted because of a sponsor's disability), the allowance for extended or continued benefits was required to be separately stated in a policy in order to guarantee coverage for employees not actively at work and for dependents who may require hospitalization; this term should be contrasted with continuation of benefits that apply after termination of employment; *see also continuation*

eye care capitation or carve out—*see vision carve out*

eye examinations—a common additional benefit for HMO coverage; *see also additional benefits to Medicare risk, and vision carve out*

F

FAcct—Foundation for Accountability; a collaboration of private and public health purchasers, including HCFA, and consumer groups working to develop outcome measures that will allow comparison of the quality of care delivered in managed care settings with those in fee-for-service settings; FAcct's purpose is to provide information about the quality of health care to purchasers and consumers

face sheet—*see discharge summary*

factored rating—*see adjusted community rating*

faculty practice plan—*see FPP*

fail safe—*see Medicare Preservation Act of 1995*

failing company defense—the legal defense used against antitrust charges involving acquisition of a failing medical company, substantiated by the theory that the acquisition does not substantially lessen competition; generally supported in court if the failing company can neither meet near-term financial obligations, nor successfully reorganize; *see also antitrust laws*

family dependent or family member—*see dependent*

favorable selection—occurs when an insurer enrolls a higher percentage of healthy, low-risk members who do not utilize as much care as the population as a whole; favorable selection has occurred in early Medicare risk contracts, possibly because sicker patients tend to stay with their current doctor rather than enroll in managed care; state and federal governments are attempting to level the playing field against favorable selection through guaranteed issue, guaranteed renewal, and portability; *see also adverse selection, guaranteed issue, guaranteed renewal, portability, and risk adjustment*

favored nations status—*see most favored nations*

Federal Employee Health Benefits Program—*see FEHBP*

federal open enrollment—providers (HMOs, PPOs) that serve federal-sector employees must conduct the yearly open enrollment according to federal regulations that call for enrollment periods of at least 30 days; the Federal Employee Health Benefits Program (FEHBP) provides a choice of nearly 400 plans nationwide to nearly 9 million covered lives, with choices of over 20–30 plans during open enrollment in some areas

federal qualification—the designation rendered by HCFA after a methodical review to determine a plan's adequate preparation to become an HMO (according to the procedures of Title XIII of the PHS Act); the business review includes a review of documentation, contracts that are required for support by individual providers or hospital systems, infrastructure systems and facilities, marketing capabilities, accountant's evidence of fiscal soundness; *see also desk review, FQHMO, and HMO Act*

Federal Trade Commission Act—*see FTC Act*

federally qualified community health center—*see FQHC*

federally qualified HMO—*see FQHMO; see also federal qualification*

fee disclosure—any discussion or communication that makes a patient aware of the charges before treatment is rendered

fee for service—*see FFS*

fee maximum—the most that a PCP may be reimbursed for any particular health care service, as contractually agreed upon as terms for participation in a plan; normally tied to a regional assessment of those fees that are usual, reasonable, or customary; *see also reasonable and customary charge*

fee schedule—under a fee-for-service arrangement, or discounted FFS, the fee schedule is the document that outlines all predetermined fee maximums that the participating provider

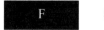

will be paid by the health plan within the period of the contract; *see also Medicare fee schedule*

fee schedule indexing—a payment mechanism for PCPs, designed to encourage them to move toward managed care, in a format that keeps the advantages of FFS, but with an index bonus or penalty, based on cost-effective care delivery; fee schedule indexing is applied to the individual PCP payment; not as good as full personal capitation; *see also FFS, and full personal capitation*

fee schedule payment area—a geographical area under Medicare for which the payment for a specified service is the same

fee splitting—an unethical "kick-back" practice of a physician, surgeon, or consultant returning part of the professional fee back to the referring physician for making the referral; fee splitting is practically ruled out under relationships of managed care in which the PCP is at risk or sharing risk with specialists

FEHB Guide—Federal Employee Health Benefits Guide; includes information about candidate health plans that seek to offer coverage to federal employees as part of the yearly enrollment period; lists 388 plans for the 1997 enrollment, including the NCQA ranking for quality; *see also federal open enrollment, and NCQA*

FEHBP—Federal Employee Health Benefits Program; a federal government health care insurance for federal employees

FFS—fee for service; the full rate of charge for a patient without any type of insurance arrangement, discounted arrangement, or prepaid health plan; before managed care this was the typical mechanism for pay for care; serious problems of cost containment under this traditional reimbursement setting included churning, and coding creep, in addition to charges that may have been excessive in relation to the actual cost of providing care or services; *see also churning, and coding creep*

FFS equivalency—a quantitative measure of the difference between the amount a physician and/or other provider receives from an alternative reimbursement system, e.g., capitation, compared to FFS

FFS incentives—when physicians are paid FFS for each item of service rendered, there is an incentive to do more work to earn more money; in some IPA settings that involve FFS payment with a portion of the fee withheld, the plan or IPA can provide tracking and measurement by physician to control utilization, which allows a return of some or all or the withhold if overall financial performance warrants; *see also neutral incentive*

FFS reimbursement—*see FFS*

FFS withhold—a reimbursement strategy that is most commonly used by network model HMOs to pay physicians, and is basically fee for service using some level or percentage of a bonus withhold, which is later paid back to the physician, depending on his or her utilization efficiency; *see fee schedule indexing*

field underwriting—occurs when a plan sends members of the sales department to the field to perform a screening with prospective buyers of the proposed products, which may include the quotation of tentative premiums for various groupings of covered lives in order to determine interest in the products, and in turn, the products' profitability

50/50 rule—an HMO or CMP cannot have more than 50% of its enrollees in either a Medicare or Medicaid combined status (to ensure a safeguard against inadequate care quality to this population); there must be one commercial patient for every federal patient in the HMO; there are waivers to the 50/50 rule for Medicare and Medicaid risk, for reasons such as the inherent populations of the market comprising an abnormally high percentage of Medicare and Medicaid eligibles, and there is some discussion of further waiver to the 50/50 rule to allow certain HMOs to focus on this segment (waiver is proposed within the Administration's draft proposal of DEC 95, based on 5 major and 8 minor areas of compliance)

first dollar coverage—an insurance plan that is constructed so that there is no deductible

fiscal intermediary—an agent or entity that has agreed to provide a variety of administrative, claims payment, consultation, and member/provider services as a liaison linking a carrier, provider, and patients; *see also Blue Cross plan, and TPA*

fiscal soundness—a key concern for policy and regulation surrounding the HMO industry; applicants as federally qualified HMOs must provide independently certified financial statements for the most recent fiscal years in the Documents section of their application to include opinion of a CPA, statement of revenues and expenses, balance sheet, statement of cash flows, explanatory notes, management letter, statements of changes in net worth; also included are recent unaudited financial statements, independently certified audited financial statements of guarantors and lenders, Annual Reports for all public corporations or subsidiaries, and a copy of the prospectus for any entity having raised capital through public offerings within the last three years

flat-rate pricing models—three types of pricing models currently used by hospitals include capitation (fixed annual fee per enrollee), per case or case rate (flat rate per admission), and per diem (flat rate per day of hospital stay)

flexible benefit plan—many employers offer a menu of options to their employees, as are suitable to their needs or their ability to pay; decisions regarding which plan is needed may be made at the time of need for service; many of these plans meet the criteria of cafeteria plans according to IRS specifications; *see also cafeteria plan, and POS plan*

flexible spending account—an employee health plan option that allows a portion of employee earnings to be deposited into an annual reserve account (currently the IRS does not allow carryover, so the reserves are "use or lose" each year) on a pretax basis, normally for full-time employees with optional family member coverage; the employee can select from a variety of health plan coverage features as allowed, including drugs, DME, dental, physical exams, eye care, hearing care, mental health, ambulance, and other expenses that may be unreimbursed from other insurance coverage; consists of a separate account for employees (Health Care Account or HCA) and family members (Dependent Care Account or DCA) subject to limits and IRS regulation; offered as a low-cost service to the employee, also provides tax savings to the employer; *see also flexible benefit plan*

foot care—a common additional benefit offered by risk HMOs; *see additional benefits to Medicare risk*

formulary—a selection of drugs chosen by a hospital or MCO for use in treating patients; drugs not included in the formulary are not used unless by exception, or unless the patient is willing to pay for an added charge; may also mandate substitution of generic drugs for brand-name drugs

Foundation for Accountability—*see FAcct*

Foundation model—a non-profit PHO-type structure that might be considered more integrated than either the GPWW, open or closed PHO, which had its genesis in markets that did not allow physicians to be directly employed by hospitals—therefore a subsidiary was formed; contains MSO centralized support and physician practice procurement features, but MSO costs are paid by the foundation, not physicians; may allow physicians to share in revenue; *see also GPWW, MSO, and PHO*

FPP—faculty practice plan; based at teaching hospitals, these group practice entities may be either a single group consisting of all physicians involved in patient care for the system, or various group practice entities for specialty care

FQHC—federally qualified community health center; a type of community health center that has received federal funding by meeting certain qualifications; overseen by the Bureau of Primary Health Care, of Health and Human Services; a growing number of FQHCs are contracting as Medicaid managed care providers—over 150 in 1994; *see also CHC*

FQHMO—federally qualified health maintenance organization; a designation given by HCFA, under Title XIII of the PHS Act for an HMO that meets all the requirements of federal qualification; *see also federal qualification*

fraud and abuse legislation—in addition to the original Social Security Act law against making false benefit claims or statements, Congress added criminal and felony treatment of kickback schemes in 1977, and in 1981 added civil penalties against providers submitting improper claims for Medicare and Medicaid, with yet broader restrictions in 1987; *see also Stark I, and Stark II*

freedom of choice—a law within some states that changes an enrollee's ability to select a source of care, depending on the perspective of the freedom of choice law; a law may allow an enrollee the right to select a non-network provider and pay no added cost within a PPO arrangement, assuming the provider accepts the PPO payment rate; or, for Medicaid, 45 states currently have freedom of choice waivers, without which Medicaid beneficiaries can be seen by any provider and are not required by the state to enroll in managed care; *see also PPO*

free-standing emergency medical service center—these centers feature expanded hours of operation at costs below traditional emergency room settings for conditions such as sore throats, sprains, and lacerations in convenient locations for the patient

free-standing health benefit—HCFA's definition for a benefit that is not integrated or incorporated into a basic health benefits package or major medical plan; is offered by a carrier other than the one offering the basic coverage; and is subject to a premium separate from that of the basic package (such as dental, optical, or prescription drug); may also be called supplemental services or additional benefits; *see also additional benefits to Medicare risk*

free-standing MSO—a management services organization that is not hospital or physician affiliated, in terms of a subsidiary or ownership relationship, but rather is developed by private investors (who could be physicians) not tied to any specific local medical society or physician network; *see also MSO, hospital affiliated, and MSO, physician affiliated*

frequency—the number of times a service was provided

FTC—Federal Trade Commission; relevant function to review mergers and acquisitions of HMOs, hospitals, medical groups, or various levels of health networks or combinations of the above entities, to ensure no infringements of anti-trust laws

FTC Act—(15 U.S.C., 45) establishes illegal declarations of unfair competition, and deceptive or unfair practices that encompass health care; has a generally broader application than either the Sherman or Clayton restrictions; *see also Clayton Act, and Sherman Act*

FTE—full-time equivalent, used to define a full-time staffing position that is devoted to a particular function

FTEP—full-time equivalent physician

full and fair disclosure—each HMO must prepare a written description of the following: benefits (including limitations and exclusions), coverage (including a statement of conditions on eligibility for benefits), procedures for obtaining and being denied benefits, rates, grievance procedures, service area, participating providers, and its financial condition including at least the following from the most recent audit—current assets, other assets, total assets, current liabilities, long liabilities, and net worth

full capitation—may be used to describe either physician capitation at the individual-physician level, or global capitation for all aspects of care; *see also full personal capitation, and global capitation*

full charges—*see FFS*

full network ownership—*see asset merger model*

full personal capitation—considered perhaps the ideal method of advanced capitation at the level of the individual PCP, who receives a PMPM to cover specialist expenses; the method can allow a PCP to become more efficient while ensuring quality of care, which in turn allows more enrollees per PCP; early use of full personal capitation may favor either the protection of the PCP from specialist risk, or catastrophic costs (i.e., above $3,750 PMPY) or may include 6–12-month moving average payments; does not include global risk for facility costs; or may also include a Medicare risk contractor that is entirely responsible for both Part A and B service costs at AAPCC rates; *see also contact capitation, downstream costs, global capitation, and PMPM*

full-risk capitation—*see global capitation*

full-service network—another name for vertically integrated networks; *see also vertical integration*

full-time student—because full-time students are allowed dependent coverage up to a certain age, a definition of their status is required for insurance purposes; a full-time student is a student who is enrolled for a sufficient number of credit hours in a semester or other academic term to enable the student to complete the course of study within not more than the number of semesters or other academic terms normally required to complete that course of study on a full-time basis at the school of enrollment

fully capitated—*see global capitation*

G

GAF—geographic adjustment factor; the average of the three geographic practice cost indexes (GPCI) for a geographic area; this measure is used to determine accurate payment within the payment areas of the Medicare fee schedule; *see also GPCI*

gag clause—the name given to a contract clause between insurers and their network physicians that restricts communication between physician and patient regarding noncovered services, or recommendations to nonnetwork providers; a current area of dispute between physicians and insurers

gatekeeper model—a managed care design in which a PCP serves as gatekeeper for the patient's initial contact for medical care and referrals; used within closed access or closed panel structures; this feature precludes the patient from obtaining care from multiple sources, and also precludes the patient from gaining unnecessary direct access to specialty care; *see also referral provider, and secondary care*

GDP—gross domestic product; a measure of our nation's total value of all goods and services produced within a year, relevant to health care programs in the sense that GDP is tied to various health care entitlement and funding mechanisms at the state or national level

generalist—a family practice provider, general internist, or general pediatrician who has not been trained as a specialist

generic drug—*see generic equivalents*

generic equivalents—drug products not protected by a trademark that have the same active chemical ingredients as those sold under proprietary brand names

geographic adjustment factor—*see GAF*

geographic area—a specific reference used by HCFA to define the service area for an HMO or CMP; the area within which the HMO or CMP furnishes, or arranges for furnishing, the full range of services that it offers to its Medicare enrollees; *see also service area*

geographic practice cost indices—*see GPCI*

geriatric outreach—a subset area of community outreach, which is any activity by providers or insurers to bring education or medical services to the elderly, particularly in cases where they lack adequate understanding of medications, medical procedures, health plan coverage, or proper access to transportation, particularly in cases of mobility limitations; may be provided through geriatric outreach coordinators, geriatric nurses, briefings, telephone assistance, or help in using a health care system that often seems complex to seniors

GHAA—Group Health Association of America, Inc.; a Washington DC-based trade group representing more than 100 managed care plans; recently joined with AMCRA and is contemplating a name change to reflect the new entity

GHI—group health insurance

global budget—a government technique of setting a total expenditure ceiling or cap for all of the nation's health care expenditures, versus regulating the price of individual fee elements

global capitation—a reimbursement mechanism that pays for all of the care needs for a population of patients, including physicians and hospitals; may involve payment from an HMO to each PCP at risk for a contractually determined PMPM amount, which is to pay for the costs of all physician services; or may involve payment to a provider network or IDN for all physician and hospital care, with other stated commitments or limitations for pharmacy, mental health, or other carve outs; a portion of the global cap may be withheld in a reserve fund to pay for specialist care referred by the PCP (excess remaining each year is paid out, or shortages are carried forward against

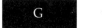

future global capitation payments to the PCP); *see also capitation, carve out, IDN, PCP, PCR, and risk*

global fee—*see package pricing; see also category-based pricing, and DRG-specific per-case pricing*

global per diem—a reimbursement mechanism used by a provider to include all costs of care for a day, fixed regardless of case type; *see also category-based pricing, and DRG-specific per-case pricing*

GPCI—geographic practice cost indices; the HCFA system used to adjust RBRVS, by calculating the cost of running a medical practice in 210 national payment areas, based on a national average; include components of work, practice, and malpractice expenses; the GPCI's validity is challenged by many physicians and analysts, who point to wide variations in payment rates and irrational geographical areas (Wisconsin has 11, but Minnesota has 1); HCFA won't change them without wide physician support, and no draft reform bill has recommended change, perhaps due to the demographics of physicians who benefit from current GPCI; *see also RBRVS*

GPWW—group practice without walls; an early managed care market structure that allows physicians to retain their separate offices, and combines centralized business operations with decentralized delivery of care in hopes to preserve traditional autonomy; comprising a group of physicians with varying interests and geographical locations, who may or may not have hospital affiliations as primary care or specialty orientations; GPWWs fail to attract meaningful covered lives; *see also management service bureau*

grace period—within the context of the enrollee paying premiums on time, contracts outline the number of days (30, 60, etc.) past the due date under which medical coverage will still be granted, assuming payment is ultimately made before the end of the grace period

graphical user interface—*see GUI*

grievance procedure—a procedure that is enumerated in the standard contract between HMO and employer/purchaser, in which a health plan member or participating provider can air complaints and seek remedies according to a chain-of-command, and requires a response within a stated period of time; procedures must ensure that grievances and complaints are transmitted in a timely manner to appropriate HMO decision makers, and that appropriate action is taken promptly (including a full investigation if necessary and notification of concerned parties as to the results)

group—the combination of subscribers receiving health coverage, as opposed to an individual who may purchase insurance; group medical coverage is provided by an employer for its employees

group boycott—any market condition involving deselection or exclusion of providers, in which the managed care organization is found guilty of anticompetitive intent, or exclusivity, and exclusion without reason upon more than one provider; *see also AWP laws, and exclusivity*

group contract—a managed care contract with a medical group rather than individual physicians; the document that includes an application for coverage, together with any additional contract clauses signed by both the health plan and the enrolling entity, which constitutes the agreement regarding benefits, exclusions, and other conditions between the health plan and the enrolling unit

group enrollment period—a period of at least 10 working days each calendar year during which each eligible employee is given the opportunity to select among the alternatives included in a health benefits plan, within the context of section 417.150 of CFR-42

group insurance—a health services contract or insurance policy that covers groups of employees, and may also include their family members, within one contract; normally provided by an employer; *see also group*

group model HMO—involves contracts between an HMO and either a single or multiple group of physicians and hospitals; the medical groups may be organized as a partnership, professional corporation, or other association; the health plan compensates the medical group for covered services at a contracted rate and arranges hospital services agreements for the inpatient or ancillary care needs; *see also IPA-HMO, network model HMO, and staff model HMO*

group practice—a combined practice of three or more physicians or dentists who share office personnel, expenses, equipment, space records, or income

group practice without walls—*see GPWW*

group purchasing—a common feature for physician management companies and IPAs to provide discounts on various supplies and services to the members, to include: medical supplies, e-mail or Internet type services, banking services, telephone or paging services, office supplies and service contracts, and malpractice insurance discounts

group-to-group portability—an increasingly popular health plan feature of legislative initiatives in the Senate and House for employees who want a guarantee that they will continue to receive coverage even after they change job or insurers, regardless of any preexisting medical conditions; *see also group-to-individual portability, and portability*

group-to-individual portability—the current draft of Senate legislation that would require insurers to offer coverage to individuals who lose their employer coverage and seek individual coverage, regardless of preexisting conditions; *see also group-to-group portability, and portability*

guaranteed issue—refers to a policy within a growing number of state laws that requires an insurer to issue insurance to any small group in the state, if they market small group coverage, regardless of preexisting conditions of any members

guaranteed renewable—*see guaranteed renewal*

guaranteed renewal—refers to a policy within a growing number of state laws that requires an insurer and health plan to renew a policy for a company or individual who was previously enrolled, as long as the premiums are continually paid

GUI—graphical user interface; the computer capability that displays a picture or image on the screen, versus only letters and numbers; commonly referred to as icons, which are clicked by the computer mouse arrow, in order to open a file, activate a command, or step through a computer program

Hart-Scott-Rodino Act—(15 U.S.C., 18a) mandates premerger notification to the FTC and the Department of Justice within this section 7A of the Clayton Act, if the acquiring entity has net sales or annual assets of more than $100 million, or if the acquired entity has net assets of $10 million, or vice versa; *see also Clayton Act*

HBA—Health Benefits Advisor; the title for a staff member in a military treatment facility who assists patients receiving their health care benefits and seeking any reimbursement according to the CHAMPUS, or a TRICARE point-of-service program of enrollment

HCA—Health Care Account; within the structure of employee flexible spending accounts that meet Internal Revenue Service criteria; employers maintain a separate account for the employees, called Health Care Accounts or HCAs (separate from the account for family members, called Dependent Care Accounts or DCAs); *see also DCA, and flexible spending account*

HCAs—hospital cooperation acts; *see COPA law*

HCF—Health Care Finder; the title given to a staff member of a provider or health plan who assists patients in obtaining referral care or diagnostic tests; used within the Department of Defense TRICARE program

HCFA—Health Care Financing Administration; the federal agency responsible for administering Medicare and overseeing states' administration of Medicaid; also reviews Medicare HMO applications and publishes reports on plan performance

HCFA 1500—a standardized claim form, developed by HCFA, for providers of services to bill professional fees to health carriers or third parties; not used for hospital or institutional charges; *see also UB-92*

HCFA Common Procedural Coding System—*see HCPCS*

HCFA physician marketing restrictions—HCFA has published a set of restrictions that define unethical behavior by physicians who may become involved in marketing managed care products, such as providing a patient with a comparative cost or benefit information between plans, sharing data from one insurer to another, and becoming directly involved in enrollment without appropriate health plan marketing involvement (insurer's materials and approach must meet advance HCFA approval before use); however, physicians may speak of the benefits of managed care or provide personal letters to patients

HCPCS—HCFA Common Procedural Coding System; a five-digit set of codes used by Medicare to describe a series of provider services, supplies, and procedures; includes CPT codes but also others that supplement CPT, such as for DME, ambulance services, and physical therapy; *see also CPT*

HCPP—Health Care Prepayment Plan; one of the three distinct types of managed care contract alternatives for Medicare members under HCFA; HCPPs under HCFA are paid by Medicare comparable to cost HMOs, but HCPPs only partially cover Medicare benefits and do not provide any of the additional benefits that risk HMOs do (such as eye glasses or prescription drugs); some HCPPs cover all Part B benefits and others cover only partially; HCPPs do not cover Part A services, but some may arrange for Part A services and file Part A claims for its members; *see also cost contract*

HCQIA—Health Care Quality Improvement Act; this federal law addresses peer review and credentialing activity that seeks to improve the quality of care, granting an immunity of quality-related functions and programs from falling under state and federal law against antitrust; *see also antitrust laws, credentialing, and PRO*

Health and Human Services—*see HHS*

Health Arizona—state legislation passed as Proposition 203 during part of the national election process in November 1996, which granted families of four or more with less than $15,000 income per year to have access to health care benefits paid by the state

health assessment—*see health risk assessment*

Health Benefits Advisor—*see HBA*

health benefits contract—a contract or other agreement between an employing entity or a designee and a carrier for the provision of, or payment for, health benefits to eligible employees or to eligible employees and their eligible dependents

health benefits package—the complete set of covered services and supplies that have been contracted between an HMO and its enrolled membership

health benefits plan—any arrangement to provide or pay for health services that is offered to eligible employees, or to eligible employees and their eligible dependents, by or on behalf of an employing entity

Health Care Account—*see HCA*

health care center for adults—*see adult day health care center*

Health Care Financing Administration—*see HCFA*

Health Care Finder—*see HCF*

Health Care Prepayment Plan—*see HCPP*

Health Care Quality Improvement Act—*see HCQIA*

health coverage—insurance to protect against the risk of sickness or injury; provides payment of benefits for medical services and supplies, dental, disability, and various other options or included benefits as listed within the contract; *see also carve out, and prepaid care*

health education—*see health promotion; see also additional benefits to Medicare risk*

health fair—an activity that is conducted either for purposes of disease prevention (which can be a service for a population already at risk with a plan or provider), community goodwill, or a marketing or consumer education effort directed toward future enrollment or future use of a medical practice, hospital, or other medical facility; health fairs include such activities as distribution of verbal and written information on self care, effective use of a medical system or plan, assistance in selection of a physician or plan (either as an individual consumer or selection from multiple employer options), and basic health screenings, such as cholesterol, blood pressure, or visual checks

health history—the medical history of a potential enrolled plan member that assists underwriting personnel in evaluating the likelihood and acceptability of medical risk

health insurance purchasing cooperative—*see HIPC*

health level seven—*see HL7*

health maintenance organization—*see HMO*

health plan—a description of any of a variety of HMOs, CMPs, PPOs, indemnity, or other legal entities that act as insurers to provide health care services to enrolled members

health plan broker—*see patient broker*

health plan data analysis—the generic field within the managed care industry that is growing in importance for the study of financial, workload, and population data for a market or product type; the core of work that yields actuariay-developed premium rates, risk decisions for potential cost and stay outliers, and negotiations between plans and providers

Health Plan Employer Data and Information Set—*see HEDIS*

health plan purchasing cooperative—*see HPPC*

health plan regulation—also called HMO regulation; legislation introduced to promote consumer protection and consumer confidence in HMOs, provide for enhanced patient claims denial appeals options, require rectification of managed care entities by an accrediting body on a given frequency (such as by NCQA every three years), and disclose physician payment methods; *see also appeals and hearings, NCQA, and unregulated provider entities*

health professional shortage area—*see HPSA*

health professionals—physicians (doctors of medicine and doctors of osteopathy), dentists, nurses, podiatrists, optometrists, physicians' assistants, clinical psychologists, social workers, pharmacists, nutritionists, occupational therapists, physical therapists, and other professionals engaged in the delivery of health services who are licensed, practice under an institutional license, are certified, or practice under authority of an HMO, a medical group, IPA, or other authority consistent with state law

health promotion—activities by an individual educator, physician, provider group, IDS, or HMO, that are oriented toward providing the patient or enrolled population with various educational materials, lectures, health risk assessments and appraisals, incentives or disincentives, or interactive discussion settings that create awareness of healthy lifestyles; teaching the population how to remain healthy and keep costs low; may include self-care and proper use of a PCP or care options; most programs include subjects such as smoking, weight control, exercise, eating habits, stress, cholesterol, and blood pressure

health purchasing alliance—*see purchasing alliance*

health purchasing cooperative—*see HIPC*

health risk assessment—a health promotion or wellness program used to evaluate the health status of a patient or employee, which can either be performed on-site or off-site from the work location, through an automated or written format of questions and answers; programs may determine either general health status or may be more targeted toward cardiovascular health, with related risks and recommendations for how to reduce risks; some plans or programs conduct an initial assessment for all members, and also conduct executive or high-stress occupation physicals, while others use a case manager for follow-up and coordination of other care needs; *see also case manager, health promotion, and wellness program*

Health Security Act—proposed by President Clinton as part of national health care reform leading up to the 1992 presidential election, the Health Security Act was not enacted, but contained HIPC-type applications of employee choice among competitive plans and insurers with standard benefit packages, standard employee contribution with optional added coverage out-of-pocket, premium capitations, government price controls, restrictions for preexisting condition limits, POS option or other out-of-network coverage, specified dental coverage for children under 18, use of common definitions and standardized data elements for collection and electronic transmission, portability, guaranteed renewals for groups, and universal access

health service agreement—*see HSA*

health status and enrollment—under HCFA guidelines, an HMO may not, on the basis of health status, health care needs, or age of the individual, expel or refuse to reenroll any enrolleeor refuse to enroll individual members of a group

health system agency—an entity that has been designated in accordance with section 1515 of the Public Health Service Act

hearing aids—a common additional benefit to members enrolled in HMOs; *see additional benefits to Medicare risk*

HEDIS—Health Plan Employer Data and Information Set; the result of a coordinated development effort by NCQA to provide a group of 60 performance measures that gives employers some objective information with which to evaluate health plans and hold them accountable; HEDIS helps ensure that plans and purchasers of care are speaking the same language when they are comparing value and accountability

HHA—home health agency; a licensed facility or program that is certified or otherwise authorized by state and federal laws, and approved by the plan to provide contract health services

HHS—Health and Human Services; an organization with nearly 200 years of history in some form since the establishment of the first Marine Hospital in 1798, but more recently established as a Cabinet-level Department of Health, Education and Welfare in 1953, under which the Medicare and Medicaid programs were created in 1965; the new Department of Health and Human Services was official on May 4, 1980; responsible for medical and social science research, preventing outbreak of infectious disease, including immunization services, ensuring food and drug safety, Medicare (health insurance for elderly and disabled Americans) and Medicaid (health insurance for low-income people), financial assistance for low-income families (AFDC), child support enforcement, improving maternal and infant health, Head Start (preschool education and services), preventing child abuse and domestic violence, substance abuse treatment and prevention, and services for older Americans, including home-delivered meals

HI—hospital insurance; also known as Medicare Part A; this program provides basic insurance against the costs of hospital and related post-hospital services for Medicare eligibles; *see Medicare Part A*

high risk—high chance of loss, including a small chance of high loss

HIPC—health insurance purchasing cooperative or coalition (or in California, Health Insurance Plan of California); often pronounced "hip-ick"; one of many types of a purchasing alliance, begun by California in 1992 without premium capitations, or state price controls; designed to spread the risk of small group and individual health care members among a broad representation of purchasers, and guarantee insurance to small businesses of 3 to 50 employees; proposed as part of national health care reform in 1992—many reform proposals surrounding President Clinton's Health Security Act also contained HIPC applications of restrictions for preexisting condition limits, portability, guaranteed renewals for groups, and universal access; acts as the purchasing agent for consumers under a system of managed competition in negotiating the best plan at the lowest cost from networks of doctors and hospitals or HMOs; *see also care system model, Health Security Act, and purchasing alliance*

HL7—health level seven; a health automation standard that contains formats and protocols for transmitting health information between systems; the HL7 message format is a substantial body of documentation that includes data element-level field descriptions for medical orders, test results, etc., for all commonly used requirements

HMO—health maintenance organization; the common name given to a line of business devoted to managing populations of patients through a prepaid premium, and selling this licensed product directly (or retail) to the employer or purchaser; the four types of HMO models are the group model, IPA, network, and staff model; under the federal HMO act, an entity must have three characteristics: an organized system for providing health care or otherwise ensuring health care delivery in a geographic area, an agreed-on set of basic and supplemental health maintenance and treatment services, and a voluntarily enrolled group of patients; *see also group model HMO, IPA-HMO, network model HMO, retail HMO, staff model HMO, and wholesale*

HMO Act—a 1973 federal act (42 U.S.C., 300 *et seq.*) outlining requirements for federal qualification of HMOs, consisting of

legal and organizational structures, financial strength requirements, marketing provisions, and health care delivery; the voluntary status of "federally qualified" is sought in order to gain
credibility with employers, and the chance to gain covered
lives from dual choice mandates that require employee access
to such plans; *see also dual choice, and federal qualification*

HMO market penetration—*see penetration rate*

HMO party in interest—*see party in interest*

HMO policymaking body—a board of directors, governing
body, or other body of individuals that has the authority to
establish policy for the HMO

hold-harmless clause—a clause in some managed care contracts
that designates who is and is not held responsible for any contractual liability; required by many state and federal regulations; often written to give the provider sole responsibility;
some states require provisions to hold patients harmless from
claims by providers, even if the insurer becomes insolvent

holding company legal model—an organizational structure normally existing before subsequent integration, in which a parent
or holding company is used over subsidiary hospitals or
groups that often perform related functions but have a distinct
corporate identity; the reason for substituting holding company format for an integrated relationship is to bring efficiencies instead of redundancies that continue to exist because of
separate corporate identity; consists of separate hospital balance sheets and income statements, loss of power in the original hospital boards, shared ownership of the parent by
hospitals

home care—provision of medical care by a health care professional at the patient's home, traditionally administered in
either a more costly hospital inpatient setting or an outpatient
setting (i.e., IV therapy or physical therapy); preferred method
of care for patients not needing hospital care, or for patients not
able to ambulate to office visits

home health agency—*see HHA*

home uterine activity monitor—*see uterine monitoring*

horizontal integration—also called specialty integration; health entities that contain multiple groupings of similar care components along the continuum of care, with financial incentives for alignment into the larger group (such as multiple hospitals, or sub-acute care facilities, long-term care, home health, or behavioral health components), are combined in a system with the purpose of increased contracting leverage or increased chances of survival due to taking economies of scale and elimination of redundant overhead staff or function; *see also horizontal merger, and vertical integration*

horizontal merger—the legal reference to horizontal integration of health entities with businesses at the same or similar market level; a review target by antitrust regulators to see if merger results would substantially reduce competition; the Department of Justice outlined antitrust safety zones, with revisions in the 1994 FTC report, "Statements of Enforcement Policy and Analytical Principles Relating to Health Care and Antitrust"; *see also antitrust laws, and horizontal integration*

hospice—a licensed or certified facility that provides specialized care of the terminally ill with an interdisciplinary team of health professionals and volunteers under the direction of the patient's personal physician, which may be in the form of support for physical, social, psychological, spiritual, or nutritional needs; hospices have inherent managed care structures of interdisciplinary team care in a central location; over one billion dollars annually comes to hospices from Medicare in per diems for routine home care, inpatient care, respite care, or continuous crisis care; *see also NHO*

hospital affiliation—the contract between a plan and one or more hospitals whereby the hospital supports the inpatient requirements that the plan has agreed to provide enrollee

hospital alliance—a voluntary formation or collaborative group-ing of two or more hospitals together as a system or network (or other looser alliances) for the purpose of competing with the strengthened negotiating position of one entity in dealing with one or more health plans for managed care contracts, and possibly reducing costs through shared services or group pur-chasing; some say that loose affiliations will not bring the strongest advantages possible—but others say that the need for tightly integrated structures should be determined solely by whether they are needed to compete effectively; *see also IDN, and local hospital system*

hospital alliance messenger contracting—in a model similar to hospital alliance single-signature contracting, a contracting messenger is identified to speak for each hospital in the alli-ance, understanding the price and conditions each is willing to accept from payers, without sharing information with other member hospitals in such a way to violate FTC laws, and with-out the use of a central contracting governance committee

hospital alliance single-signature contracting—within the hos-pital alliance structure, some members form a central contract-ing governance committee to determine policies and strategies for capitated pricing requirements, resulting in the identifica-tion of a single contract specialist who is authorized to sign within stipulated boundaries; however, the FTC disallows price-fixing for other than capitated contracting by an alliance (consult an attorney for guidance); *see also messenger model*

hospital-based physician—a physician who provides services in a hospital setting and who has a contractual relationship with the hospital, such as a salaried employee; contractual relation-ships vary widely, from paying a physician an agreed amount or an agreed portion of the collections from patients, or the hospital may collect the funds from patients either in its own right or as an agent for the physician

hospital capitation—a payment arrangement for hospitals by insurers on a per-member basis, for a given number of patients under a provider's care; used as an alternative to fee-for-service, per diem, case rate, or other methods, in an effort to decouple higher payment with higher utilization; few hospitals currently are successful in obtaining capitated arrangements; without creative arrangements within the payment equation, such as the sharing of variable cost risk pool funds with the hospital, it is often not financially rewarding for hospitals to reduce utilization; *see also capitation, case rate, FFS, and hospital variable cost risk pool*

hospital contracting alliance—a group of health care purchasers that may be private, public, or combinations of both, brought together with a purpose of gaining preferred contract pricing; *see hospital alliance*

hospital cooperation act—*see COPA law*

hospital DRG risk pool—a modification of the hospital standard risk pool based on DRGs or bundled case rates, established to further enhance the hospital's incentive for utilization savings through a shared bonus distribution; similar to the hospital variable cost risk pool, but based on the estimated cost per case versus the incremental cost per day; *see also bundled case rate, case rate, hospital incremental cost of care, hospital standard risk pool, and hospital variable cost risk pool*

hospital incremental cost of care—above the level of fixed costs that a hospital needs to recover, it expends incremental amounts of money in relation to the actual costs of services and supplies for patients as they are treated; these incremental costs are the focus of new hospital capitation strategies—particularly the cost segments that are within the hospital's utilization discretion to some degree; *see also hospital DRG risk pool, hospital standard risk pool, hospital variable cost risk pool*

hospital insurance—*see HI*

hospital risk pool—any variety of risk pools established to provide a bonus distribution from hospital care savings; may be based on reimbursement methods to include case rate, DFFS, per diem, hospital standard risk pool, or hospital variable cost

risk pool; *see also case rate, DFFS, hospital standard risk pool, hospital variable cost risk pool, and per diem*

hospital spot marketing—similar to hospitals charging a fee-for-service rate for a bed day or particular hospital service; however, in this case, hospitals compete by selling the beds or services as a commodity to either physician groups, IDNs, or insurers, hoping to increase occupancy volume, but often forced to take radical cost cuts due to oversupply and competition

hospital standard risk pool—a hospital risk pool method that is established to provide a bonus distribution to the hospital from its help with utilization savings; hospitals that are unsatisfied with payment below the previous FFS method may pursue variable cost tactics; *see also capitation, and hospital variable cost risk pool*

hospital subcapitation—a subordinate capitation arrangement, in which a hospital agrees to be paid a monthly fee for a stated package of inpatient services, which are a subset of global responsibilities of a primary contract provider entity and an insurer; some subcapitation agreements allow risk pool sharing with the subcapitated facility, designed to shelter the primary contractor and incentivize the subcapitated facility toward lowered utilization; used as an alternative to per diem contracts between two providers

hospital variable cost risk pool—a risk sharing strategy (normally between a hospital and an affiliated medical group) that provides an incentive for the hospital to reduce utilization through the receipt of a bonus pool share of savings to offset lost revenue; first, the hospital performs a budget projection that includes fixed costs that must be covered for break-even by the medical group as a payment floor; then, as care is provided during the contract, the hospital is allowed payment for the actual incremental costs of inpatient care per day provided (above fixed cost); and finally, any surplus is shared according to agreement; *see also hospital incremental cost of care*

hospitalization coverage—the elements of hospital care that are included under a particular health plan; the primary consideration of patients selecting an HMO, even more important than which hospital is included in the network

HPO—Hospital–Physician Organization; a term infrequently used to describe a Physician–Hospital Organization, by virtue of the initiative coming from the hospital to form the single entity, instead of an initiative led by physicians; *see also PHO*

HPPC—health plan purchasing cooperative; *see purchasing alliance*

HPSA—health professional shortage area; any area that has a shortage of health professionals, in that the providers earn a bonus payment; the area may be either rural or urban area that is recognized by the Secretary of HHS to be underserved; *see also HHS, and rural area*

HSA—health service agreement; the description of contract benefits and associated procedures that is given to each participating employer and serves as the foundation for policy on enrollment, eligibility, termination procedures, coordination of benefits, continuation and conversion, exclusions and limitations, and general provisions; *see also COB, continuum of care, and enrollment*

hybrid—the name given to a number of blended formations for health care systems, services, plans, or products; such as a point of service hybrid plan that blends opportunities for enrolled members to choose either an HMO network or an indemnity approach for out-of-network providers; also used to describe the alternate HMO models of physician–hospital organizations, management services organizations, and integrated delivery systems; *see IDS, MSO, PHO, and POS plan*

hybrid per diem—a reimbursement arrangement made by a hospital or provider system to an HMO that takes multiple per diem categories, such as medical/surgical, obstetrics, and critical care, and blends them into a more general pricing, with the assumption that on the average, payment will be acceptable as long as the populations projected match experience for that population, and billing will be simplified; often stop losses are used for protection, when applying hybrid per diems

IBNR—incurred but not reported; represents revenue for a hospital or system that has a float type of accounting; contracts deal with IBNR, and may commit terms for this financial value of care by placing a certain amount of money in the provider's account as recognition that care has already been rendered (although there is increasing pressure by HMOs to delete these reserves); may also refer to PCP referrals to specialists; care has been provided but the carrier has not received the claim yet; the carrier sets aside IBNR reserves to allow for the projected level of future liabilities during the lag period; *see also lag study*

ICD–9 (International Classification of Diseases)—International Classification of Diseases 9th Revision; a statistical classification system consisting of a listing of diagnoses and identifying codes for reporting diagnosis of health plan enrollees identified by physicians; coding and terminology to accurately describe primary and secondary diagnosis and provide for consistent documentation for claims; the codes are revised periodically by the World Health Organization; since the Medicare Catastrophic Coverage Act of 1988, ICD–9 is mandatory for Medicare claims

ICF—intermediate care facility; a preferred, lower-cost setting within the managed care environment for patients who require only an intermediate degree of care, without hospital or skilled nursing facility capabilities, but above that of assisted living center; *see also assisted living center, and continuum of care*

identification card—a card that is issued by an HMO or other health plan entity to identify each enrollee as being eligible, according to the contract coverage agreement

IDN—integrated delivery network; commonly used instead of integrated delivery system, but may also be used when referring more to the network of providers versus the system as a whole; for example, a hospital-based IDS without an HMO license may reach agreement for its network to contract with an HMO and serve as participating provider resource for the HMO

IDS—integrated delivery system; a single organization or a group of affiliated organizations that provides the full range of health care services to a population of enrollees within a market area or fairly large regional area, which consists of physicians, dispersed clinic settings, hospitals, a referral network, and full continuum of after-care offerings; an IDS may obtain an HMO license and "retail" health services, or may "wholesale" the provision of care services and seek to accept risk within components of the systems, such as a physician network or for its hospitals, or may obtain global risk agreements with HMOs; *see also health plan, and ODS*

IHDN—Integrated Health Delivery Network; *see IDN*

IHO—integrated health organization; a single entity serving as an integrated delivery network that is fully responsible for obtaining and managing payer contracts, assuming health care risk, collecting revenue, and asset control by lease or ownership; because of these specific features it is listed separately from IDN or PHO; *see also IDN, and PHO*

immunizations—a common additional benefit to members of an HMO; *see also additional benefits to Medicare risk*

in-area—any area within the region defined by the HMO as its service area; *see also out-of-area*

in-area services—allowed and covered treatment or services that are received within the authorized service area and geographical boundaries, and provided by the plan's participating provider; *see also out-of-area, and out-of-network*

inclusive contracting—providing an opportunity to a large number of health care entities, in order to build a network or provide a service, such as an insurer developing a broad panel health plan or a large employer allowing a large number of insurers to be listed on a menu from which employees may select their preferred HMO; the desire for freedom of choice has caused the pendulum to slowly begin a swing toward inclusive plans, versus the exclusivity in earlier arrangements; *see also broad panel health plan, exclusivity, and freedom of choice*

incremental cost of care—*see hospital incremental cost of care*

incurred—the time at which medically necessary service, supplies, or treatment is rendered by a provider to a member

incurred but not reported—*see IBNR*

incurred claims—legitimate claims against the carrier that will result in expenditures to offset revenue, and become a part of the medical loss ratio against the particular product within a specified period; adjustments are normally made on a monthly basis to reflect IBNR that are ultimately received; *see also IBNR*

incurred claims loss ratio—*see MLR*

indemnify—to cover a loss

indemnity—literally, the insurance protection against injury or loss of health; although this type of traditional system is now being replaced with other forms of insurance that share risk with providers or employers, indemnity programs still exist to a large extent to provide reimbursement to the enrolled members for benefits under the contract; indemnity systems reimburse on a FFS basis for care and services

indemnity benefit contract—a contract that covers some or all of the actual expenses of providing covered services, but not more than the actual charges for a specific service; an indemnity benefit contract allows the patient to choose the doctor or hospital desired, versus being limited to providers within a panel or limited network; *see also exclusivity, FFS, and network model HMO*

indemnity carrier—usually an insurance company that offers selected coverage within a framework of fee schedules, limitation, and exclusions to coverage, as negotiated with subscriber groups; beneficiaries are reimbursed after carriers review and process filed claims

indemnity plan—*see indemnity, and indemnity benefit contract*

independent living center—*see retirement residence; see also assisted living center*

independent medical examiner—physicians who make examinations of candidates to receive disability, other than the attending physician

independent physician association—*see IPA-HMO*

independent practice association—*see IPA-HMO*

independent provider association—*see IPA-HMO*

indigent—condition of having insufficient income or savings to pay for adequate medical care without depriving oneself or dependents of food, clothing, shelter, and other essentials of living; *see also medically underserved population*

indirect costs—also called overhead costs; costs that all services share in, and are not attributable to any one business activity—versus direct costs; examples include utilities, administration, and maintenance

individual insurance—policies that provide protection to the policyholder and family; sometimes called personal insurance versus group insurance

individual network model HMO or plan—*see network model HMO*

individual practice association—*see IPA-HMO*

individual specialist capitation—a problematic method of capitated payment to specialists, comprised of the selection of specific physicians for each specialty area, and payment of a capitated amount, times the number of enrollees in the plan; individual capitation can create geographical problems of referral distance for patients and their unfamiliarity of specialists, and the plan has limited flexibility in channeling to "special expertise" specialists; also, a large number of lives is needed to sustain a specialist, yet actuarial risk may be excessive; *see also contact capitation, and specialty department capitation*

individualized incentives—used in similar references to full personal capitation, but may involve capitation for small groups, or pod-level units, or individuals; capitation for primary care services with target setting or incentives to reduce specialist referrals and inpatient care; typically, PCPs are not at risk for mental health or diagnostic services; profits and losses are shared among all PCPs; *see also full personal capitation*

information systems—managed care information systems requirements have undergone significant growth, requiring robust architecture to handle: claims processing and payment, membership enrollment, benefit management by plan/product/level, UR/UM, billing and accounts receivable and administrative support; used to track, measure, analyze, and improve performance of managed care; *see also all categories under MIS*

initial eligibility period—related to allowing early enrolling members the opportunity to apply for coverage without showing any physical examination proof of health status to the health plan, assuming they apply within the stated time frame; may be viewed as either an incentive for recruitment or the right of employees to obtain coverage by virtue of their employment

injury—any physical wound, harm, or damage to an enrollee; within the context of disability claims for worker's compensation, the focus is upon this injury coming as a result of employment; *see also disability, and disability income insurance*

inpatient—an enrollee who has been admitted to an acute hospital or other nonambulatory setting and placed under the care of a physician for at least 24 hours

inpatient days per thousand—*see days per thousand*

inpatient nonavailability statement (INAS)—certification from a military treatment facility that cannot provide medical inpatient care, allowing medical coverage to be provided at a civilian facility

inpatient physician—a physician who performs primary or exclusive responsibilities for inpatients, to include the admissions from other primary care physicians, in order to bring the benefits of an "inpatient expert provider" to the patient, and to the financial performance results that come from enhanced utilization practices, internal hospital procedures, coordination with case management or discharge planning, or other streamlining; performs patient rounds, coordinates ICU transfers, seeks improved hospital efficiencies, and ensures discharge planning requirements; often performed by an internal medicine physician or family practitioner; *see also CM, and discharge planning*

insolvency conditions—agreements between parties such as plans and reinsurance entities automatically terminate on the date of the HMO's insolvency—this is why the federal government is so careful in defining the qualifications for an HMO; insolvency is a determination by a court of competent jurisdiction that is made at a point that forces all operations of the plan (or the reinsurer) to cease, and occurs on the date of the court declaration; operations are not considered ceased as long as the plan is under control of a receiver until the receiver stops paying for future services, declares its intention to not make payments, and orders the plan providers to stop rendering services on behalf of the plan, other than services for which they have already been paid

insurable risk—the conditions that make a risk insurable are: the peril must produce a definite loss not under the control of the insured; many others are subject to the peril; the loss is quanti-fiable and the cost of insurance is feasible; and the peril must be unlikely to affect all insured simultaneously

insured—any person or organization qualifying as an insured under a contract or policy, for benefits according to the policy that are received in return for payment

insurer–provider alliance or partnership—*see ODS—second definition*

integrated call management—an important strategy to improve speed and efficiency in many health care applications through the use of multiple automated system components for telesystems support or medical information systems design; characterized by an open information systems architecture, which allows an organization to develop or add to systems that have been selected for their compatibility with a wide variety of other instruments or technology; automated call sequencers, call screen transfer capability, and voice response systems are only components within an integrated call management system; *see also call screen transfer capability, open information systems architecture, and voice response system*

integrated clinical program—a collaboration of health care practitioner, provider, and payer entities who share in the risk and reward for cost-effective, high-quality care for a defined population

integrated delivery network—*see IDN*

integrated delivery system—*see IDS*

integrated health delivery network—*see IHDN*

integrated health organization—*see IHO*

integration—the organizational construction of a health care entity that may consist of various affiliated organizations at differing levels of the care continuum, with the purpose of providing the best possible health care for patients; emphasis on the importance of "economic hand-off" interactions between levels (i.e., subacute versus traditional hospitalization) and prudent utilization at the appropriate level; also features an optimum linkage and interaction among all segments in the system, for shared efficiencies when possible; *see also continuum of care*

intensity of service—*see volume and intensity of service*

intent to deny—if HCFA finds that an entity does not appear to meet the requirements for HMO qualification but appears to be able to meet them within 60 days, it issues a notice of intent to deny, with a summary of the basis for the finding; within 60 days from the date of notice, the entity may respond in writing to the issues, and may revise its application to remedy any defects; *see also denial and reconsideration*

intermediary risk—occurs with the sharing or transfer of risk from an insurer to an intermediary entity, such as an integrated delivery network, a hospital, physician, IPA, or physician group; with the sharing or transfer of risk comes the potential to share or transfer the profits associated with efficient care operations

intermediate care facility—*see ICF*

internal case manager—a medical professional (usually a nurse), whose primary case management function is to follow certain types of seriously ill, high-risk, or surgical patients in the hospital to ensure that their progress is monitored and that they are moved to the least expensive care alternative as soon as appropriate; internal case managers have achieved remarkable results in reducing length of stay, ICU, and step-down costs; *see also case manager, and CM*

International Classification of Diseases—*see ICD–9*

Internet services—*see on-line services*

IP—inpatient

IPA-HMO (individual practice association; independent physician association; independent practice association; independent provider association)—physicians form a separate legal entity, usually a corporation or partnership, which contracts with the payer/HMO to arrange care in private offices through individual contracts with member physicians in return for a negotiated fee; the IPA in turn contracts with physicians who continue in their existing individual or group practices; the individual practice association may compensate the physicians on a per capita, fee schedule, or FFS basis; represents a wholesale health care delivery component (working with a payer/HMO/retailer that markets the plan directly to employers or patients); *see also HMO*

job lock—an employment phenomenon that occurs whenever an employee feels locked into a current job, because of the attending fear of not being able to get health insurance from a subsequent employer, particularly due to a preexisting medical condition; *see also portability*

Joint Commission—Joint Commission on Accreditation of Healthcare Organizations, formerly JCAH (Joint Commission on Accreditation of Hospitals); an accreditation body for clinics, hospitals, home care, other medical facilities, and health networks; the seal of approval by this nonprofit agency is the goal of most for-profit, public, and even federal or military facilities, and its approval may be contractually mandated by HMOs for network hospitals; recently expanded criteria include Malcolm Baldridge quality standards and other managed care guidelines for health plans; *see also NCQA*

joint contracting model—an alliance between an integrated care system and a physician organization to provide effective, high-quality care within the most cost-efficient setting; *see IDS*

joint marketing—the marketing of health care coverage or services, performed jointly by an insurer and provider, to highlight the individual and combined strength or brand identity of the partners; joint marketing is made more effective by the sharing of information between insurer and provider that can provide mutual "win-win" outcomes, such as unique insight on a market advantage that would benefit from publicity, patients needing case management, or prospective managed care enrollees

joint venture (JV)—arrangement involving risk and benefit sharing between one or more other entities, with rights and obligations specified in contractual terms, for a specific purpose;

examples include a hospital JV with a provider group for 50% of the group profits or "downside" risk, a hospital JV with an HMO for 50% exposure to the mutual patient business, or a hospital buying a certain percent of common shares of an HMO together with other terms that encourage broadened sharing of business

K

Kassebaum-Kennedy Health Coverage Bill—the name of legislation passed in August 1996, which began on July 1, 1997; the
bill primarily benefits those who already have insurance but
suddenly lose or change jobs, and also benefits the self-
employed or employees of small businesses, and those who
leave jobs with insurance and want to buy an individual policy; portability and fixed premiums are guaranteed for those
who change jobs, as long as they have been insured for 12
months (regardless of whether they quit, are fired, or are laid
off); options consist of high and low coverage alternatives; also
provides tax deductions for the chronic or terminally ill; no
help for 40 million Americans currently without insurance;
allows insurers to sell 750,000 high deductible policies between
1997 and 2000, with deductibles between $1,500 and 2,250
($3,000–4,500) per person (per family) followed by opening an
MSA, which is tax free from contributions and earnings but
capped at 65% (75%) of the deductible per person (per family)
per year; *see also MSA, and portability*

key management staff—within the context of applying for status
as a federally qualified HMO under DHHS/HCFA procedures
(as well as the standard requirement for bidding other
employer or government business), the HMO must indicate
which individuals are responsible for key management functions, what percent of time they spend toward the HMO, and
by whom they are employed (for the categories of executive,
medical, UR, finance, marketing, Medicare coordinator, management information systems, and other)

L

lag factor—the key accounting factor within a lag study, relating to IBNR claims that have been incurred but not received or processed for payment in the months following the close of a particular accounting period; *see also lag study and IBNR*

lag study—a report that tells HMO management how old their claims are at the point of being processed, monthly payments for the current month and past months, and monthly accruals toward expenses

LAN—local area network; information technology used within health care and other industries to connect multiple user workstations to a single communications network that allows shared access to file servers or other tools; LANs allow valuable information sharing from one workstation to any other station on the network; various configurations of "rings" or "star" networks have been developed to connect the workstations; *see also wireless technology*

lapse—termination of insurance due to nonpayment of premium in time

least restrictive level of care—care levels vary in cost and intensity, all the way from once-a-week outpatient care to inpatient care; the managed care standard calls for the least restrictive level of care that offers sufficient safety and effective treatment at the least cost, within the continuum of all possible care alternatives

legacy system—computer hardware or software applications that do not have the features of open systems architecture or easy integration with other systems; legacy systems are either replaced entirely or slowly moved toward a future central system within the system strategic planning process for a health system or information systems entity

legal reserve—the minimum reserve that a company must keep to meet future claims and obligations as they are calculated under state code

length of stay—*see ALOS*

length of stay legislation—in cases where safeguards against substandard care may need to be imposed so that patients are not discharged until it is medically appropriate, such as for mothers and infants after childbirth, legislation is being introduced that would set a minimum length of stay, i.e., at 48 hours for vaginal delivery and 96 hours following a Caesarean section; the opposition states that clinical decision making should be free of politics

level premium—rating structure in which the premium level remains the same throughout the life of the policy

liability protection—HCFA requires each HMO to adopt and maintain satisfactory arrangements to protect its enrollees from incurring liability for any fees belonging to the HMO, and precludes balance billing; liability protection can be obtained through insurance, financial reserves held against insolvency, and other means acceptable to HCFA

lifetime disability benefit—disability income provision payable for an insured's lifetime as long as the insured is totally disabled

limited charge—the Medicare fee limit amount, specified by legislation and based on the par fee, that nonparticipating providers may charge above the fee schedule

limited duty—any work assignment given to temporarily disabled employees that is limited in scope (no heavy lifting or prolonged walking) and time (three weeks)

limited liability company or corporation—*see LLC*

limited policy—policy that covers only specified accidents or sicknesses

limiting charge policy—a policy implemented in 1993 to ensure that nonparticipating physicians are not allowed to charge more than 115% of the Medicare-allowable charge; *see also balance billing, and nonparticipating provider*

LLC—limited liability company or corporation; a legal entity that provides for partnership agreements, liability protection of the owners, entering into contracts by the owners or designee(s), and an excellent way to share risk and equity between hospital systems and physician practices; an LLC has the advantage of a corporation but is taxed as a partnership, therefore it is an ideal vehicle for a joint venture between a nonprofit and a for-profit

local area network—*see LAN*

local hospital system—in the context of multihospital systems configurations or integrated hospital systems, a local hospital system is characterized by having one or more hospitals in an urban area (the flagship entity) and at least one added hospital somewhere within a 60-mile radius; *see also hospital alliance*

locality—*see fee schedule payment area*

lock-in—primarily used to describe a patient's obligation to use an HMO's participating provider in order to receive payment for covered services according to the benefit plan, rather than using out-of-network providers who have not agreed to give a discount to the payer or patient; considered to be a key to reducing costs in HMOs versus PPOs; *see also covered services, enrollment lock-in period, out-of-network, POS plan, and PPO*

longitudinal patient record—a patient record that is structured to include the documentation of care provided from all past sites of care during a given period, versus keeping separate records at each primary care site or hospitalization location with no ability for centralized access of the medical information; the growth of automation to support medicine has brought a focus toward longitudinal records within networks or local systems of care

long-term care—*see LTC*

long-term care insurance—the principal insurance provision that gives patients a freedom from concern about bankruptcy or the catastrophic impacts of long-term care

long-term disability income insurance—within the context of replacing income, this insurance benefit helps replace earned income lost through a disability

long-term disability insurance—a provision to pay benefits to a covered person as long as he or she remains disabled, up to a specified period exceeding two years

LOS—length of stay; *see ALOS*

loss—eligible expenses under an agreement that are actually incurred on behalf of members during the contract year and paid by the plan during the contract year or the three-month period immediately following the contract; loss does not include: claim administration expenses or salaries paid to employees of the plan; any amount paid by the plan for punitive, exemplary, extra contractual, or compensatory damages awarded or paid to any member arising out of the handling, investigation, litigation, or settlement of any claim; or failure to pay or delay in payment of any plan benefits, or any statutory penalty imposed upon the plan on account of any unfair trade practice or any unfair claim practice; or amounts paid by the plan after the three-month period following the contract year without the express written approval of the reinsurer

loss ratio—*see MLR*

low volume DRGs—DRGs with five or fewer patients in a hospital's base year

loyal hospital contract strategy—the reverse of a loyal physician contract strategy, in which the physicians affiliated with a hospital use their market strength to ensure a payer accepts the hospital into the contract (because of their loyalty to the hospital system)—or else the physicians will not become part of the network for the payer; *see also loyal physician contract strategy*

loyal physician contract strategy—the practice by a hospital system and its affiliated physicians of establishing unity when negotiating with payers, so that they are not picked apart for the payers' preferred segments of the system; the strategy is effected by creation of a joint venture for contracts, and insertion of a contract clause that commits the payers to offer the "all or nothing" contracts to the hospital and physicians; legal entity binding hospital to physicians may be a PHO or MSO; *see also HPO, loyal hospital contract strategy, MSO, and PHO*

LTC—long-term care; the segment of the health care continuum that consists of maintenance, custodial, and health services for the chronically ill or disabled; may be provided on an inpatient (rehabilitation facility, nursing home, mental hospital) or outpatient basis, or at home; *see also assisted living center, continuum of care, and rehabilitation facility*

MA—*see market area*

MAC list—maximum allowable charge or cost list; relates to the basic maximum allowance of pharmaceuticals, normally stated at the generic level, for provision within a plan; the network pharmacies within a plan must adhere to this listing, together with any updates or modifications; *see also AWP*

mail-order drug program—a growing number of HMOs affiliated with corporations or federal contracts use mail-order drug programs to ensure their members have timely access to discount rate drugs

major diagnostic category—*see MDC*

major medical expense insurance—a form of health insurance that provides benefits for most types of medical expense up to a high maximum benefit; may contain internal limits and is usually subject to deductibles and coinsurance

malpractice expense—the incurred cost of malpractice insurance, defined as one of three specific components within the relative value scale; *see also RVS*

malpractice insurance—insurance that protects providers against loss incurred as the result of litigation expenses or judgments for damages resulting from allegations or findings of failure of the provider to use due care in the conduct of a professional service; IPAs, physician management corporations, or large hospital systems can typically get reduced rates for malpractice insurance through volume discounts

managed behavioral care—mental health or chemical dependency treatment that is screened and monitored for meeting utilization criteria, treatment effectiveness, and/or quality

managed care—any method of health care delivery designed to reduce unnecessary utilization of services, and provide for cost containment while ensuring that high quality of care or performance is maintained; a system to minimize cost of care and "churning" while still delivering good access to high-quality health care; arrangements made by payers to promote cost-effective health care through establishing selective relationships with health care providers, developing coordinated or integrated delivery systems, and conducting medical management activities; *see also managed health care plan*

managed care organization—*see MCO*

managed competition—used to describe a proposed system that generally provides for universal coverage, employer contribution of a fixed sum for the employee's plan of choice, with transferable coverage between jobs, designed to discourage unnecessary utilization by the patient, and the conscientious selection of care plans (who would also be offering their most competitive rates); premium rates are not community rated or tied to any specific employer age-sex derivations, but blended broadly across the United States; this concept was drafted by the "Jackson Hole Group"

managed health care plan—one or more products that integrate financing and management with the delivery of health care services to an enrolled population; an employer, purchaser, or insurance company contracts with either individual providers or an organized provider network that delivers services and may share financial risk or have some incentive to deliver quality, cost-effective services; the health care plan uses or contracts the services of an information system capable of monitoring costs and evaluating patterns of members' use of medical services

managed indemnity—an indemnity-type health insurance program or style of health care delivery that features some type of reimbursement mechanism to encourage lowering the utilization of care by patients, beyond the method of pure indemnity, but less than at-risk contracting or more advanced integration strategies; may include a bonus or withhold pool used with a discounted FFS, or some degree of physicians becoming organized; *see also DFFS, fee schedule indexing, and indemnity*

management information systems—*see MIS*

management service bureau—an early stage of managed care MSO structure to support physicians' practices, provided by a subsidiary of the local hospital to bring cost efficiencies through centralized billing services, group purchasing, personnel management, and other menu options; it costs little to create and allows rapid network growth while retaining physician independence, but accomplishes little in terms of meaningful long-term loyalty of physicians or protection from payer network lock-out; *see also MSO*

management services organization—*see MSO*

mandated benefits—*see clinical mandate*

mandatory point-of-service—the legal requirement for an eligible organization contracting as a PPO to mandatorily offer its enrollees a POS option; there is a growing interest at the state and federal level to commit legislation of this type, to include the Clinton administration's current (Dec 95) draft of Medicare policy; *see also POS plan*

manual rates—claims rates that are constructed from the average claims of a carrier, with adjustments for the particular characteristics of various industries, groups, or plans

market area—geographic region for a carrier's primary market; may include some of the same descriptions as service area, but market area may overlap service area

market pressure—often a primary determinant for decisions by a provider or health plan regarding what levels of benefits or types of services to offer, as a competitive response to what other plans are providing—assuming competitive forces exist between two or more providers or health plans; *see also community standard*

market share—defined as a percent of the potential market within an area that involves competition among plans, for either FFS, PPO, or HMO business

marketing directory—*see physician referral service*

marketing ethics violations—the government seeks to protect enrollees in Medicaid and Medicare managed care programs from becoming the targets of unethical marketing and recruitment—hence the review of marketing approach and strategy before and after granting federal qualification; health plans have been charged with lying to enrollees, bribing them, and going door to door to influence enrollment decisions through various means

marketing Medicare—HCFA review—*see Medicare marketing*

master group contract—a legal document between the enrolling unit and the carrier, setting forth in detail the rights and obligations of the enrolling unit, covered person and carrier, and terms of the coverage

master patient index—*see MPI*

master person index—*see MPI*

Maternal and Child Health Programs (MCHP)—a state service organization to assist children under 21 years of age who have conditions leading to health problems

maternity length of stay legislation—in 1995, a debate captured national attention regarding what the minimum mandatory length of stay should be following childbirth, in response to the American College of Obstetricians' concerns that many mothers were being prematurely discharged, within 48 hours of delivery, in the interests of reducing costs under managed care;

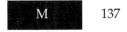

five states enacted legislation and 31 more states had legislation pending in 1996; *see also anti–managed care legislation*

maximum allowable cost list—*see MAC list*

maximum out-of-pocket costs—the limit on total member copayments, deductibles, and co-insurance under a benefit contract; sometimes health plans will specify that copays are excluded from consideration

MCO—managed care organization; a generic term applied to a managed care plan; also called HMO, PPO, EPO, although the MCO may not conform exactly to any of these formats

MCR—modified community rating; *see CRC*

MDC—major diagnostic category; a grouping of diagnoses by major organ systems, using the ICD-9 codes; valuable for utilization or cost analyses and reports that are less detailed than the actual DRG; *see also DRG, and ICD–9*

means testing—*see Medicare affluence testing*

Measure 44—state legislation in Oregon that was passed by a 55% to 45% margin as part of the national election of November 1996, bringing added revenue to the state's Medicaid program called the Oregon Health Plan, by increasing cigarette tax by 30 cents per pack; a portion of the revenue will also fund smoking cessation programs

MECA—Medicare Expanded Choice Act; *see Medicare Choices demonstration project*

Medicaid—a medical program of aid provided by the federal government and administered at the state level to provide preventive, acute, and long-term benefits with little or no patient cost share, with benefits according to established criteria for the poor, aged, blind and disabled, and aid to dependent children; current legislative proposals would provide block grants to the states, or other strategies to make them responsible for the program with less dependence on the federal level; the federal government matches state spending through grants on a sliding scale for per capita income; California and New York also require local government contributions for the state

Medicaid Section 1115 waiver—allows the state an exemption to administering Medicaid in accordance with Section 1115, with an alternate Medicaid managed care demonstration or model that is applied statewide; granted by HCFA in order to speed the implementation savings of managed care in the states, while possibly discovering an improved methodology; *see also Medicaid Section 1915(b) waiver*

Medicaid Section 1915(b) waiver—allows a state to perform an alternate Medicaid managed care demonstration or model at the local level, or on a regional or state basis; *see also Medicaid Section 1115 waiver*

Medicaid state matching rate—current legislative proposals for Medicaid reform involving block grants to the state, involving a state matching rate of 1:1, or even a one dollar federal contribution matched with 80 cents from the state, as in the National Governors' Association plan; *see also block grant*

Medi-Cal—the California version of the Medicaid federally aided, state-operated and administered program that provides medical benefits for certain low-income persons in need

medical care evaluation—the component of a quality assurance program that looks at the process of providing quality medical care

medical diagnostic category—one of a set of categories of mutually exclusive principal diagnosis areas that correspond to a single body system or etiology, and in general are associated with a particular medical specialty

medical director—physician, usually employed by a hospital or health plan, who services in a medical and administrative capacity as head of the organized medical staff or key approval authority for referral and hospitalization decisions, and may have subordinate staff performing case management, utilization management, or quality of care disciplines

medical group—any partnership, association, or group of three or more physicians, dentists, psychologists, podiatrists, or other licensed health care providers working together in medical practice; some group practices pool their income and use a portion of it to employ staff, provide for shared equipment, facilities, common records, or may also use a portion of their income to distribute among members or retain profits to build the group's net worth; the effect of managed care upon managed care group profitability has been mostly bipolar—those who do not choose managed care may be left behind in gaining the new efficiency skills, only to see the value of their groups decline, while the other groups that become successful in adapting to managed care will remain profitable and may remain independent while adding and training other physicians to the group or pod-level formations

medical group incentive—by placing a medical group or pod-level group at risk to some degree, incentives are created among the physicians to control utilization of outpatient and inpatient services, referrals, diagnostic procedures, pharmacy, and other downstream costs; many medical group incentive strategies involve a withhold; *see also neutral incentives, and PCR*

medical group member—a health professional engaged as a partner, associate, or shareholder in the medical group; or any other health professional employed by the group who may be designated as a medical group member by the medical group

Medical Group Practice—*see medical group*

medical incidents—any act or omission in the furnishing of professional health care services; any such act or omission, together with all related acts or omissions in the furnishing of such services to any one person, is considered one medical incident

medical loss ratio—*see MLR*

medical protocols—also called best practices, critical and clinical pathways, clinical algorithms, practice guidelines or practice parameters; guidelines that result from clinical trials as the currently accepted best way to prevent, detect, or treat a medical condition; guidelines that insurance plans or MCO may require physicians to follow in order to be part of their panel; provide specific treatment options or steps to follow when a provider sees a patient with a particular set of clinical symptoms or lab data; *see also diagnosis protocols, prevention protocols, and treatment protocols*

Medical Quality Commission—a nonprofit accreditation authority, whose charitable mission since 1991 includes setting standards for prepaid health plans, with three-year certificates for medical groups and IPAs on a full or provisional basis; also conducts research and structures programs for outcomes, case management, quality, risk, and utilization management; *see also Joint Commission, NCQA, and URAC*

medical record—record of a patient maintained by a hospital or a physician for the purpose of documenting clinical data on diagnosis, treatment, and outcome

medical record administrator—person who maintains records that meet the medical, administrative, legal, ethical, regulatory, and institutional requirements of a hospital

medical savings account—*see MSA*

medical services organization—used to describe either a management services organization (MSO) or physician management corporation (PMC)

medical staff organization—an organization of physicians within a group of hospitals that seek to contract for health care services, but do not necessarily contract with the hospital (as does the PHO); *see also PHO*

medical staff–hospital organization—*see PHO*

medical underwriting—*see underwriting*

medically indigent—persons in need of financial assistance and/or whose income and personal resources will not allow them to pay for costs of care

medically necessary—the litmus test of whether health care treatment is warranted, judged against consistency between the diagnosis, medical documentation, and the likelihood that peers within the medical community accept the treatment as necessary for the patient

medically underserved area—a significant definition, in that federally qualified HMOs, which show within their application a projected enrollment of at least 30% of its members from a medically underserved population when the HMO first receives financial assistance or becomes operational, must identify the area in which that population resides, the total population of that area, and the percent of anticipated enrollment to be drawn from the area; *see also medically underserved population*

medically underserved population—the population of an urban or rural area as described in section 417.912(d) of 42 Code of Federal Regulation, Chapter IV, to include the ratio of primary care physicians to population, the infant mortality rate, the percent of population age 65 and over, the percent of population with family income below the poverty level, and with the designation by the Secretary of DHHS; *see also indigent*

Medicare—a national program of health insurance that has been operated by HCFA on behalf of the federal government since its creation by Title XVIII—Health Insurance for the Aged in 1965 as an amendment to the Social Security Act, which provides health insurance benefits primarily to persons over the age of 65 and others who are eligible for Social Security benefits, and covers the cost of hospitalization, medical care, and some related services; Part A includes inpatient costs and Part B includes outpatient costs

Medicare affluence testing—a formula, procedure, or policy that would increase Medicare FFS premiums for those with higher income, after testing the financial means of beneficiaries to determine ability to pay; considered by a July 95 House Ways & Means Subcommittee on Health; the draft Medicare Preservation Act approach would charge higher premiums to single seniors with incomes over $75,000 and couples with incomes over $125,000, with elimination of subsidy at $100,000 for singles and $150,000 for couples (citing Congressional Budget Office estimates for a 65-year-old couple, retiring this year, who will take out $126,000 more from Medicare than they paid in during their working years)

Medicare arrangement—a written agreement executed between an HMO or CMP and another entity in which the other entity agrees to furnish specified services to Medicare enrollees of the HMO or CMP, but the HMO or CMP retains responsibility for those services; Medicare payment to the HMO or CMP discharges the beneficiary's obligation to pay for the service

Medicare beneficiary—*see QMB*

Medicare cost contract—*see cost contract*

Medicare Economic Index—*see MEI*

Medicare eligible—*see QMB*

Medicare enrollee—the specific reference to an enrollee, member, or subscriber that is given by HCFA to mean an individual who is entitled to Medicare benefits (Part A and Part B or Part B only) and who has been identified on HCFA records as an enrollee of an HMO or CMP that has a contract under section 1876 of the Act; *see also new Medicare enrollee*

Medicare fee schedule—a payment schedule used by Medicare to pay for physician services, based on the amount of resources consumed in providing the care, referred to as the RBRVS; replaced the Customary, Prevailing, and Reasonable Charge (CPR) method; *see RBRVS; see also CPR*

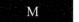

Medicare marketing prohibitions—in offering its plan to Medicare beneficiaries, an HMO or CMP may not: discriminate (for example, recruit high income only), mislead or confuse (i.e., "our plan is recommended by HCFA"), offer gifts or payment as an inducement to enroll, perform door-to-door solicitation, or distribute marketing materials known to be disapproved by HCFA; *see also HCFA physician marketing restrictions*

Medicare marketing–HCFA review—HCFA reviews applications from prospective Medicare managed care health plans to ensure they include an overall marketing approach, advertising/promotion strategy, plans for community education and public relations, marketing staffing, and the marketing budget; marketing activities must provide potential Medicare enrollees with adequate written descriptions of the additional benefits or services, or reductions in premiums, deductible, or copays that may pertain under risk reimbursement; *see also federal qualification*

Medicare marketing–physician steering—efforts by a physician, normally the direct consultation of a physician with a Medicare eligible patient upon the conclusion of an office visit, which allows the physician to share verbal and written benefits of participating in a managed care plan (with the physician serving as the primary care manager); an effective recruitment tool for physicians to add to their Medicare panel, within the limits of Medicare marketing prohibitions; *see HCFA physician marketing restrictions, Medicare marketing prohibitions, and Medicare marketing-social recruitment*

Medicare marketing–social recruitment—a Medicare enrollment marketing and recruitment strategy that is designed to offer an appealing setting for senior citizens, such as a local restaurant (also called "pie meetings"), where members of a provider, medical group, or health plan present a briefing that outlines the benefits of joining the recruiter's managed care plan; physicians and existing managed care patients are influential speakers at these social events; *see also Medicare open house recruitment, and telemarketing*

Medicare/Medicaid case—refers to an individual who receives medical and/or disability benefits from both Medicare and Medicaid; also called Medi-Medi case

Medicare open house recruitment—a Medicare enrollment marketing and recruitment strategy that is designed to give the prospective member an opportunity to come into the recruiter's facility in order to receive written and verbal information about the provider, medical group, or health plan, and thereby gain a positive impression from the host's capability to provide service, and favorably influence the senior citizen's enrollment decision

Medicare Part A—an insurance program (also called Hospital Insurance program) that provides basic protection against the costs of hospital and related post-hospital services for: individuals age 65 or over and eligible for retirement benefits under the Social Security or the Railroad Retirement System, individuals under age 65 entitled to not less than 24 months of benefits under the Social Security or Railroad Retirement System on the basis of disability, and certain other individuals with end stage renal disease and covered by the Social Security or Railroad Retirement System; after various cost sharing requirements are met, Part A pays for inpatient hospital, skilled nursing facility (SNF), and home health care; the Hospital Insurance program is financed from a separate trust fund, primarily funded with a payroll tax levied on employers, employees, and the self-employed; *see also Medicare*

Medicare Part B—supplementary Medical Insurance Program, which is a voluntary portion of Medicare, and includes physicians' services to all enrollees who are willing to pay a monthly premium, and are also entitled to Medicare Part A; *see also Medicare*

Medicare Part B premium share—the portion of Part B paid by the patient was designed in 1965 to be one-half of the program costs; in 1974 Congress limited increases to Social Security COLA equivalents, and as costs increased, the premiums fell below 25% of costs; in 1984 Congress said that premiums

would continue at 25%; the 1990 OBRA preset premiums from 1991–1995 based on estimates at 25% each year; but the 1995 premium of $46.10 was 31.5% of program cost, so the 1993 OBRA returned to a 25% beginning in FY96; the FY96 budget reconciliation bill proposed freezing the contribution at 31.5%, to save $44 billion in seven years, with affluence testing; *see also COLA, Medicare affluence testing, Medicare Preservation Act of 1995, and OBRA*

Medicare Payment Review Commission—*see MPRC*

Medicare Plus—the name given to one draft alternative to traditional Medicare (not to be confused with MediChoice), which was outlined in the Medicare Preservation Act of November 1995 and also in the congressional budget reconciliation bill (H.R. 2491), featuring the beneficiary's choice of any plan available where they live, to include FFS, coordinated care through HMOs, PPOs, POS plans, and PSNs, a $6,000 deductible plan with a medical savings account, union or association plans; the congressional budget office predicted savings of $27 billion if 24% enrolled by 2002; *see also Medicare Preservation Act of 1995, and MediChoice*

Medicare+Choice—legislation in which Medicare expanded the number of eligible private and public entity risk contractors, as part of the Balanced Budget Act of 1997 in which current HMOs and CMPs are automatically transitioned but must comply with new rules, while PSOs also are allowed to accept Medicare risk; applications to become a Medicare+Choice demonstration site first began in 1995 as a way to encourage metropolitan areas with high numbers of Medicare eligibles, yet low percentages of Medicare HMO penetration, to develop new HMO constructs (and to test the receptivity of beneficiaries to enroll in a broad range of options) to help reduce health care costs; Medicare+Choice plans must be state licensed as risk-bearing entities except those PSOs that obtain three-year federal waivers from state licensure; *see also Balanced Budget Act of 1997, demonstration project, and PSO*

Medicare Preservation Act of 1995—introduced by the House Republican leadership as a plan to preserve, protect, and strengthen Medicare, and maintain its solvency in the face of projected bankruptcy by 2002; consisted of six components to: keep our government's commitment to traditional Medicare; allow seniors the same choices as others; root out waste, fraud, and abuse; maximize the taxpayer's health care dollar; test the affluence for taxpayer subsidized premiums; and guarantee the solvency through a budgetary "fail safe" provision (or annual check by the Secretary of HHS to ensure spending doesn't exceed funding)

Medicare rebate—proposed as a federal provision to allow a Medicare enrollee to make a tax-free deposit into a medical savings account, from any proceeds that come as a result of obtaining managed care from a plan that offers a premium that is lower than the monthly Medicare payment, or to use the money to purchase added benefits, assuming the enrollee did not participate in the high deductible MSA; *see also MSA*

Medicare risk—the generic name given to either the product or classification of managed care delivery in support of any of the HCFA-sponsored programs that involve an element of risk, providing care for members age 65 and older; a Medicare managed care contracting basis used in contrast to the previous fee-for-service cost contracting; Medicare risk contracts are presently used by 9% of eligibles, and some studies show that HCFA's risk contract costs to date have increased due to favorable selection by HMOs; *see also favorable selection, federal qualification, Medicare arrangement, and Medicare Choices demonstration project*

Medicare risk contract—*see Medicare risk*

Medicare SELECT—a type of Medigap insurance plan that often limits coverage to a limited or select panel of participating providers, plus the allowance of emergency and out-of-area care; *see also Medigap (MG) policy, OOA, and participating provider*

Medicare senior advisor or representative—a Medicare support advisor, preferably selected from the ranks of its enrolled members, to provide membership services, and serve as a liaison to aid in retention of members for the provider, medical group, or health plan

Medicare subvention for military retirees—provisions within the Balanced Budget Act of 1997 allowed the Department of Defense to conduct a 3-year Medicare risk demonstration project for military retirees treated within military treatment facilities; the selected sites were Keesler Air Force Base in Biloxi, MS; Wilford Hall Air Force Medical Center and Brooke Army Medical Center in San Antonio, TX; Sheppard Air Force Base in Wichita Falls, TX; Fort Sill in Lawton, OK; Fort Carson and the Air Force Academy in Colorado Springs, CO; Naval Medical Center San Diego in San Diego, CA; Madigan Army Medical Center in Fort Lewis, WA; and Dover Air Force Base in Dover, DE; previously these retirees were treated only on a space-available basis within military treatment facilities, and frequently space was not available

Medicare supplement policy—a plan that pays for the component of health care services that Medicare does not pay for, as a supplement to other care desired by the patient; a variety of commercial insurance entities are involved in this market, providing coverage for the member's coinsurance, deductible and copayments, or other added benefits; these supplements are called MediSup, Medigap, Medicare wrap, or wraparound supplements

Medicare trust fund—Medicare Part A is funded from payroll tax contributions—this fund has received much recent discussion regarding its 2002 deficit projection, as hospital insurance costs have outpaced revenue contributions; Part B is funded on a yearly basis with a percentage shared by beneficiary and the federal government; this has varied since 1965 (see Medicare Part B premium share), but is currently at 75% for government and 25% for beneficiary

Medicare Volume Performance Standard—*see MVPS*

MediChoice—a Medicare Plus type of draft plan from July 1995 of the House Ways & Means Subcommittee on Health, which features incentives to use Medicare risk, an opening for PPOs and other hybrid plans to provide care, and a defined contribution to the plan of choice (but not negotiable vouchers for individual health shopping); not to be confused with Medicare Plus; *see also Medicare Plus*

Medigap policy—*see MG policy*

MediGrant—a proposed block grant given by the federal government to the states as the only federal assistance for Medicaid; after this grant, the remaining responsibility rests with the state: to provide Medicaid benefits for pregnant women and children to age 13 with incomes up to 100% of federal poverty level, to provide coverage of the disabled (as defined by the states), to define medical assistance (under which few benefits are mandated), and set aside funds for the elderly, disabled, low-income families, and Medicare/MediGrant dual eligibles; *see also Medicaid, and set aside*

MediSave—the name given to the Medicare Plus program medical savings account, drafted with the Medicare Preservation Act of 1995; *see MSA*

MEI—Medicare Economic Index; a measurement of the annual growth in physicians' practice costs and the general inflation associated with operating a physician practice; used as the basis for updating the Medicare volume performance standard; *see also MVPS, prevailing charge, SGR, and volume performance standard*

member—*see enrollee*

member category or member type—one of a group of classification break-downs by either age groups for pediatric or adult, or the eligibility to receive Medicare, which is tied to the structure that determines physician pay

member grievance procedure—*see grievance procedure*

member lock-in—*see lock-in*

member month—the count that includes member counts and retro (retroactive) adds and deletes, resulting in one month in which one member is enrolled

member retention—*see patient retention*

member services—an HMO, IDN, or medical group will often establish a member services department, and offer specific functions to support its enrolled members, which assists in the critical business consideration of patient retention; member services may include support for individual problems, response to questions, written, telephonic, and computer support systems, with further specialization to handle claims research, enrollment research, and common problems

member services retention bonus—*see patient retention bonus program*

members per year—the basic measure of the number of annualized members enrolled in a health plan; total member months divided by 12 months

membership service agreement—those formal understandings or contractual agreements approved by the state where the plan agrees to provide the services described in the certificate of coverage issued to plan members; may also include the applicable membership service agreements that have been previously reviewed and approved by the reinsurer

mental health carve out—within the amount of PMPM that is contracted to meet all patient care needs, a mental health carve out often exists for specified services of mental health or substance abuse that can be provided more efficiently through either a focused effort or separate entity contract; an example includes $1.75 to $2.50 PMPM for annual benefits of 30 inpatient days and 20 visits, with varying copay and deductible, which may include UM for: preauthorization, concurrent review, retrospective review, discharge planning, and CM

MeSH—Medical staff-hospital organization; *see PHO*

messenger model—the nickname for an early model of physician integration, normally fostered by a supporting hospital entity to help local physicians move toward more sophisticated managed care; this formation "becomes the messenger" to other nonaffiliated physicians and insurers that capabilities are being enhanced to manage care and accept risk; typically the membership is easy to obtain and very inexpensive; *see also open PHO*

messenger model hospital contracting—*see hospital alliance messenger contracting*

MET—multiple employer trust; a legal trust established by a plan sponsor that brings together a number of small, unrelated employers for the purpose of providing group medical care coverage on an insured or self-funded basis

metric—some measure of cost, quality of care, utilization of health care services, or access that is used to measure the delivery of health care; metrics that compare similar types of organizations can be valuable in reducing variation according to the quality improvement concept, and can also allow the various entities being compared to learn from best practices or medical protocols; *see also medical protocols, and QI*

metropolitan statistical area—*see MSA*

MEWA—multiple employer welfare association; a group of employers who band together for purposes of purchasing group health insurance, often through a self-funded approach to avoid state mandates and insurance regulation; MEWAs allow small employers to obtain cost-effective health coverage, assuming they have the resources to withstand the risk

MG policy—Medigap policy; a specialized insurance policy for a Medicare beneficiary that covers the "gap" of deductible and copayment amounts typically not covered under the main Medicare policy, written by a nongovernmental third-party payer; also called MedSup Medifill, or wraparound plan

midlevel practitioner or provider—physicians' assistants, clinical nurse practitioners, nurse midwives, nutritionists, aides, medical technicians, physical therapists, etc., who deliver medical care as nonphysicians, generally under the supervision of a physician, but at less cost; this group does not include physicians, dentists, optometrists, chiropractors, podiatrists, and nurses

MIG—medically insured group

military treatment facility—*see MTF*

minimum group—the fewest number of employees permitted under a state law to constitute a group for insurance purposes; the purpose of minimum group is to maintain a distinction between individual and group insurance

minimum wage—the applicability of health plan coverage and employment status includes a consideration of minimum wage status; during any calendar quarter of the preceding calendar year, the employer was required to pay the minimum wage specified in section 6, Fair Labor Standards Act of 1938

MIS—management information system(s) that consist of computer hardware and software to support accounting and decision-making report generation; an integral part of the ability of a plan or provider delivery system to better manage care

MIS—administrative support—this module with a managed care information system must handle a minimum of: general correspondence capability, COB and Medicare, and document tracking

MIS—benefit management—this module with a managed care information system must handle a minimum of: multiple plans, products, and levels within those respective plans and products; tracking defined benefits and events; and benefit limits by service or dollar

MIS—billing and accounts receivable—this module with a managed care information system must handle a minimum of:

structure by rate and contract type, and the amount of assignment by subscriber

MIS—claims processing and payment—this module with a managed care information system must handle a minimum of: tracking of claims and payment to the authorization, benefits, eligibility, and premiums or capitations paid; match with diagnosis, procedure, location, and service codes; capitation with allowance of FFS for multiple models; calculation of payments and benefits; routine edits, such as duplicate payment, or age/sex; EOB; multiple risk or withhold options, PPO processing and TPA fund management; and claim check payment capabilities

MIS—member enrollment—this module with a managed care information system must handle a minimum of: who is enrolled, the patient transaction history, and patient's multiple assignment (such as IPA and PHO)

MIS—UR/UM—this module with a managed care information system must handle a minimum of: each authorization or referral—by provider, protocol, or benefit level; utilization and rate for each contracted entity, provider, and type of treatment; and the patterns of treatment by provider

miscellaneous expense—expense connected with hospital insurance; hospital charges other than room and board, such as X-rays, drugs, laboratory fees, and other ancillary charges

mixed model—a managed care plan that mixes two or more types of delivery systems, such as an HMO with a closed and open panel system; may be called hybrid model

MLP—*see midlevel practitioner*

MLR—medical loss ratio; a common way of describing the efficiency of a given HMO or plan, which is a basic ratio of how much it costs to provide health benefits, versus how much revenue is made from premiums (or total medical expenses of paid claims plus the IBNR component, divided by premium revenue); medical loss ratios are being reduced during the decade of the 1990s, from the low 90% to mid-70% range, but the pendulum may be swinging back up as profitability is challenged

mobile medical equipment—medical land vehicle (including any machinery or apparatus attached thereto), whether or not self-propelled: not subject to motor vehicle registration; maintained for use exclusively on premises owned by or rented to the insured, including the ways immediately adjoining

modified community rating—*see community rating by class; see also experience rating*

modified FFS—a reimbursement mechanism that essentially pays providers on a fee-for-service basis, but with certain fee maximums established by procedure; distinct from a discounted FFS in that it may not always be the same percentage discount from the prevailing FFS; this unit-of-service type arrangement is actually a typical reimbursement mechanism for many arrangements that are considered to involve managed care, but have not evolved to global risk yet, may involve a PCR withhold; *see also DFFS, FFS, global capitation, and PCR*

morbidity—the prevalence and rate of disease within a given region, or for a stated population

mortality—death rate; the prevalence of death at each age based on previous actual experience for a given population or persons with a particular region

most favored nations—a reimbursement mechanism between an insurer and either a provider or provider group, which states essentially that any time the provider gives a better price to a second or subsequent insurer or patient, it will also notify the first insurer and give the same price reductions

MPI—master patient index or master person index; an automated information system listing of patients, which includes various standardized data elements required to identify the patient for eligibility purposes, as well as to store other codes for enrollment status within a plan, such as social security number, provider number, and date of birth; *see also CPR*

MPRC—Medicare Payment Review Commission; a proposed payment formula advisory commission outlined within a draft House bill for a balanced budget, which would review aspects of the Medicare Plus program, the fee for service program, and the effect of payment policies on health care delivery; *see also PPRC, and ProPAC*

MSA—medical savings account; the Medicare Plus proposal by the Republic leadership in 1995 offered an MSA (MediSave) option to all seniors; a senior choosing MediSave would get a high-deductible insurance policy along with a cash deposit in a medical savings account that would cover a significant portion of the deductible; the high-deductible policy would have no copays, so that seniors would be assured a limit on their out-of-pocket costs; this plan is designed to incentivize the patient to save unnecessary care expenses, yet give the patient control to spend for whatever needs may exist or to purchase long-term insurance; four states have passed bills to put MSAs into Medicaid pilots, with 38 others considering bills in 1995; the Kassebaum-Kennedy bill granted the first MSAs; *see also Kassebaum-Kennedy Health Coverage Bill*

MSA—metropolitan statistical area; normally the entire metropolitan area surrounding a major city, having the characteristics of relatively close economic ties to the nucleus of the city; often the best representation for data, versus a city, county, or state

MSO—management services organization; a legal entity offering practice management and administrative support to physicians, or may purchase physician practices and obtain payer contracts as a PHO; can be a wholly owned, for-profit subsidiary of a hospital, a hospital–physician joint venture, or a private joint venture with physicians or hospital/physicians; offers a menu of services (group purchasing discounts, practice management, consulting, information newsletters and educational seminars, computer/information systems, marketing, employee leasing for office coverage, claims processing), through shared practice management; creates economies and allows physicians to delegate management and administration, but yields some profit for these functions; corporate examples include Coastal, InPhyNet, MedPartners, and PhyCor; also called physician practice management or physician management corporations; *see also PHO*

MSO, hospital affiliated—an MSO that functions as a for-profit subsidiary of a sponsoring hospital; *see also MSO*

MSO, physician affiliated—an MSO that is owned by a physician group; *see also MSO*

MTF—military treatment facility; one of any of the uniformed services medical centers, hospitals, or clinics; also called military hospitals or military clinics

multidisciplinary care plan—a treatment plan that centers around a single patient, using the expertise of a sufficiently large variety of medical specialists, depending upon the medical condition of the patient

multiple employer trust—*see MET*

multiple option plan—*see dual choice*

multiprovider network—*see IDN, and PPO*

multispecialty group practice—a group of providers, in which at least one physician is either a family practitioner, internist, or general medical officer and the others practice other specialties

MVPS—Medicare Volume Performance Standard; a spending goal for Medicare Part B services, established by Congress or by a statutory default formula that links to the Medicare Economic Index (MEI), or the annual growth in physicians' practice costs; the MVPS has a two-year delay between the year of data reviewed and the year of update; *see also MEI*

NAIC—National Association of Insurance Commissioners; national trade association with no official policy authority, which promotes cooperation and communication between the state insurance regulators (who in turn are charged with regulating the insurance industry and providing uniformity for approval and policy of HMOs within their respective states)

NAS—nonavailability statement; within the CHAMPUS system, a nonavailability statement must be issued to constitute referral approval whenever an MTF can't provide the inpatient care (or 1 of about 20 costly diagnostic or outpatient procedures) but lives within the MTF's "catchment" area of financial responsibility; the NAS consent statement is signed by the hospital commander in order to approve nonemergency inpatient care at a civilian hospital

National Association of Insurance Commissioners—*see NAIC*

national claims history system—*see NCH*

National Committee for Quality Assurance—*see NCQA*

national drug code—*see NDC*

national health care reform—*see Health Security Act*

national health insurance—often refers to a federally funded and regulated system, such as the system in Canada, but does not necessarily include federal funding and regulation; any system that would provide all Americans access to an agreed-on standard of health care

National Hospice Organization—*see NHO*

National Hospital Discharge Survey—*see NHDS*

National Practitioner Data Bank—*see NPDB*

NCH—national claims history system; originated in 1991 as the common file that combines Part A and Part B claims data for the Health Care Financing Administration; *see also HCFA, Medicare Part A, and Medicare Part B*

NCQA—National Committee for Quality Assurance; an independent, private-sector group that was jointly formed by AMCRA and GHAA in 1979 to promote QA, standards, performance measures, review procedures of HMOs and similar types of plans, and render an accreditation; a team of surveyors is sent to review an HMO quality assurance program for days—thoroughly reviewing everything from the credentialing process to recordkeeping; NCQA is becoming a hallmark of quality for an HMO (working cooperatively with leading American corporations), and it is estimated that nearly half of all HMOs have now submitted their operations for review, assuming they have been providing comprehensive services through a defined delivery system for at least 18 months; *see also AAAHC, CHAP, Joint Commission, and URAC*

NCQA Report Card Pilot Project—an effort involving managed care organizations, employer-purchasers, consumers, and union representatives in developing comparative reports on a core set of HEDIS measures

NCQA standards—include guidance or program review of: written credentialing and renewal policies, the conduct of initial and periodic review and approval of those procedures, credentials committee or PRO designation, the actual credentialing for all practitioners, DEA compliance for controlled substances, verification of malpractice coverage, liability claims history, board certification or graduate medical school verification, work history, status of good standing at any admitting facility, personal statements of competency, NPDB checks, any appraisal documentation, site reviews of practitioners, statements of delegated activities, and procedures to suspend, reduce, or terminate a practitioner with reports and appeals options; *see also credentialing, and NPDB*

NDC—national drug code; a national classification system for identification of drugs

NEC—not elsewhere classified; used in ICD-9-CM when the coder lacks the information necessary to code the term in a more specific way

negotiating alliance—*see purchasing alliance*

net loss ratio—HMOs calculate this ratio of claims and miscellaneous expenses, over premium revenues; the ratio includes accounting for all expenses, versus the medical loss ratio cost of only medical claim expenses; *see also medical loss ratio*

network capitation model—the description for any type of global capitation arrangement between a payer and a provider network; the network could be an IDN, MSO, PHO, or any formation of hospital(s) and physician(s) entities to accept the primary risk for a member population and thereby receive the capitated PMPM payment from the payer; the network must agree to governance and decision-making arrangements, since it does not have ownership or employee relationships with physicians, as does the system capitation model; network capitation requires sophisticated information systems support and extensive contracting coordination by the network entity, in order to track and pay for other subcontract relationships; *see also global capitation, hospital subcapitation, IDN, MSO, partnership capitation model, PHO, and system capitation model*

network model HMO—an HMO that involves contracts with multiple physician groups and hospitals to provide an adequate network for enrolled members; may involve contracts with large single specialty and multi-specialty groups, and also individual physicians; *see also group model HMO, IPA-HMO, and staff model HMO*

neutral incentive—generic term to define the type of payment arrangement with a physician that does not provide financial incentive for altering the pattern of care, such as the FFS incentive of churning; most staff model HMOs provide a straight salary to physicians as employees and do not provide financial motivations for more productivity (although it could be argued that by controlling utilization, physicians can help in profitability, which will ensure healthy salaries); *see also FFS incentives, medical group incentive, and pod-level risk pool*

new Medicare enrollee—a Medicare enrollee who: enrolls with an HMO or CMP after the date on which the HMO or CMP first enters into a risk contract under subpart L of CFR-42; is entitled to both Part A and Part B or Part B only at the time of enrollment; and was not enrolled with the HMO or CMP at the time he or she became entitled to benefits under Part A or eligible to enroll in Part B

new member orientation—once a member has made the decision to enroll in a managed care plan, an orientation may be given to offer service information and options for various outpatient, acute care, or urgent care that can preclude the patient's unnecessary use of the emergency room, or other high cost services; early and effective orientation of new members is seen as a key to member retention and cost savings; depending on geographical distances between members services staff and enrollees, and whether the primary focus is senior care or commercial, patient retention programs plan early one-on-one or group sessions with enrollees to aid understanding of care resources and retention; *see also patient retention*

NHDS—National Hospital Discharge Survey; a normative data source, consisting of a continuous survey that produces normative values under U.S. Census Bureau auspices, based on a sample of medical records of patients discharged from a national sample of nonfederal short stay hospitals, representing 0.8% of annual discharges; the NHDS gives insight into utilization; *see also normative data source*

NHO—National Hospice Organization; started in 1978 as a nonprofit, charitable organization that works to influence health

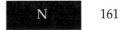

programs and public policies on hospice care and advocates the needs of the terminally ill and their families; NHO has published voluntary "Standards of a Hospice Program of Care" to outline values and principles, but does not serve as an external review entity; *see also hospice*

niche product—used to describe specialty products such as Medicare or Medicaid risk, versus commercial coverage

niche service—used to describe specialty firms in the managed care market that take carve outs or other specialty continuum of care services as their main line of business, such as dental, behavioral, or home health

nominal value—*see relative value method*

nonavailability statement—*see NAS*

noncancellable policy—also called guaranteed renewable; gives the insured the right to continue in force to a specified age such as 65, or in the case of a policy issued after age 44, for at least five years from its date of issue, by virtue of the insured's making timely payment of premiums

noncompete agreement—a legal contract clause, normally between two parties such as a provider and an insurer (but also between two insurers or two providers or other combinations) that outlines the legal commitment not to compete against each other in a particular manner; in some cases noncompete agreements are required because contract partners know significant pricing information or a confidential business strategy that could be used against the partner; some providers agree not to compete against insurers during a specific period

noncontributory—in the sense that employees do not contribute visibly toward the price of the premium, because the entire portion is paid by the employer; it could be argued that some wage and salary structures include a consideration that lower pay is a result of the employer's contribution for elements such as health care premiums

noncontributory plan—group insurance plan under which the employer does not require employees to share in its cost

nondisabling injury—an injury that may require medical care but does not result in the loss of working time or income

non-HIPC marketing—in California, which has utilized the Health Insurance Plan of California (HIPC) since 1992 as a purchasing cooperative, the participating health plans are also allowed to provide insurance to other members who are not enrolled through the HIPC projects, but their community rating must be matched for HIPC and non-HIPC business to prevent favorable selection within the non-HIPC market; *see also favorable selection, and HIPC*

nonmetropolitan area—each application to become a federally qualified HMO that projects or evidences an enrollment of at least 66% from a nonmetropolitan area must identify the area and indicate the percent of anticipated enrollment to be drawn from that area

nonoccupational policy—policy that provides coverage only for non-job-related accidents or sicknesses not covered under any workers' compensation law

nonpar—*see nonparticipating provider*

nonparticipating physician—*see nonparticipating provider*

nonparticipating provider—a provider who has not agreed to accept the rates, terms, and conditions of the health plan for treatment of the plan's enrolled members, or who does not accept the allowable charge for a plan as the full payment (whether the plan is CHAMPUS, Medicare, or another health plan); payment goes directly to the patient in this case, and the patient must pay the bill in full; the limiting charge policy ultimately determines the patient's responsibility due to balance billing; *see also balance billing, and limiting charge policy*

nonphysician practitioner—*see NPP*

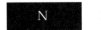

nonprofessional provider—sometimes used to describe a midlevel practitioner, or nonphysician provider; *see midlevel practitioner*

nonprofit insurers—corporations organized under special state laws to provide medical benefits on a not-for-profit basis (BCBS and Dental Service Corporations)

normative data source—one of several different kinds of data sources that are used for comparison purposes for various kinds of inpatient workload data within an institution; such as average length of stay, medical treatment days by age group, discharge rates, and DRGs; *see also ALOS, and DRG*

NOS—not otherwise specified; used in ICD-9

novation agreement—a document executed and signed by the current owner of an HMO or CMP, the proposed new owner, and HCFA or other similar entity having an arrangement with an HMO or CMP, under which HCFA recognizes the new owner as the successor in interest to the current owner's contract

NPDB—National Practitioner Data Bank; an entity with a database that is a resource for previous physician discipline or malpractice payment experience; mandatory for query by HMOs and also sought by private and federal hospitals or health systems, and even required for query by some state laws; an early step toward credentialing a provider for clinical privileges or granting status as medical director or medical staff positions; requery of NPDB is required at a two-year interval for reappointment; *see also credentialing*

NPP—nonphysician practitioner; a health care provider who is not a physician, such as a physician assistant or nurse practitioner

nurse hotline or triage system—*see telephone triage system*

nursing facility or nursing home—a segment within the long-term care facility spectrum that is oriented toward the non-acute, inpatient setting for continued care; a specially qualified facility that has the staff and equipment to provide skilled nursing care and related services for patients who need medical or nursing care or rehabilitation services; *see also SNF*

OA—open access; generally defines the ease of patient access versus the type of HMO model; open access allows the patient to select a provider of specialty care without going through a gatekeeper or primary care provider, as long as the specialist participates in the network; commonly used in the IPA-HMO; *see also IPA-HMO, and open-ended HMO*

OBRA—Omnibus Budget Reconciliation Act; what Congress calls the many annual tax and budget reconciliation acts, most of which contain language impacting managed care, or Medicare

observation unit—a health care setting that can support certain types of patients who come primarily from the emergency department (and from other clinics or outpatient settings) by providing some of the benefits of an inpatient acute bed, but without the cost; provides all-day access to a physician, with nurse observation to care for "rule-out" myocardial infarction, IV hydration, asthma, etc.; *see also transitional bed*

ODS—organized delivery system; used within the context of integrated delivery system discussions as a late transitional stage from a multihospital system toward a truly integrated network stage or ODS—first used to describe a coordinated range of services involving physicians, hospitals, and after-care to defined populations; it has more recently been used to reference alliances between insurers and providers, such as the Iowa and Nebraska models, which tie medical management strategies with the assumption of risk for a seamless system; *see also IDS*

office visit—the cognitive primary care office setting that involves examination of, or education and discussion with the patient; also used to define the event or setting for the provision of medical services other than physician services; arguably an underpaid health care setting that was the focus of RBRVS in attempting to achieve a better equality between the office visit and other procedural, surgical, or diagnostic services; *see also RBRVS*

OHI—other health insurance; health care coverage for CHAMPUS beneficiaries through an employer, an association, a dependent school coverage, or a private insurer; other health insurance must pay before CHAMPUS

ONAS—outpatient nonavailability statement; needed as authorization from an MTF commander to approve certain outpatient procedures that cannot be provided within the MTF

one-stop hospital contracting—*see hospital alliance single-signature contracting*

on-line medical record—*see EMR*

on-line services—with the growth of interactive network, or computer on-line web services, there are new ways to provide marketing and education to health care consumers; home pages or Web sites can be used to show any information previously shared by written, radio, or visual media, such as: customized directories of individual or network providers to include location maps, open enrollment information, health tips, products and services, health promotion, or even patient appointment scheduling; the future may allow member enrollment and clinical protocol data reference

on-site documentation—used in reference to the materials that must be available at the HCFA site visit to review federally qualified HMOs, including: authorization/referral forms for commercial and Medicare, encounter forms, policy manual of procedures for health professionals, long-range quality assurance plan for the HMO, minutes of UR and QA committee, and evidence that institutional providers are certified under Titles XVIII or XIX of the Social Security Act

OOA—out-of-area; the treatment obtained by a covered person outside the network service area, as defined in the contract; an area (where health care services or supplies may be received) outside the region defined by the HMO as its service area, where only emergency services are allowed; *see also in-area*

OOP—out-of-pocket; the cost of health treatment or services that must be paid by the patient, which includes coinsurance, copayment, and deductible amounts; *see also coinsurance, and deductible*

OP—outpatient; a person who receives health care services without being admitted to a hospital

open access—*see OA*

open-ended HMO—*see POS plan; see also OA*

open enrollment health fair—*see health fair*

open enrollment period—the time allowed for health plan candidates to choose a plan, either by re-enrolling in their existing plan or by switching to a competitor's plan; open enrollments are at least 30 days long and provide for a first-come, first-served basis to the limit of the plan's capacity, usually without evidence of insurability or waiting periods; most managed care plans divide member enrollment, with a major thrust in the fall for an effective date of January 1, and a minor enrollment effective July 1; *see also federal open enrollment*

open house enrollment—an enrollment marketing and recruitment strategy that is designed to give the prospective member an opportunity to come into the recruiter's facility in order to receive written and verbal information about the provider, medical group, or health plan, and thereby gain a positive impression from the host's capability to provide service, and favorably influence an enrollment decision; *see also health fair*

open information systems architecture—an important element of medical information systems design, which allows an organization to develop or add to systems that have been selected for their compatibility with a wide variety of other instruments or technology; a valuable consideration for member services or customer service operations; precludes spending money on systems that are not compatible with future expansion requirements; an example is connection of an automated telephone call sequencer, with a voice response system, and call screen transfer capability; *see also call screen transfer capability, and voice response system*

open panel—*see open access*

open PHO—an early stage managed care physician hospital organization with an open and almost nonrestrictive policy for allowing physicians to join, in an attempt to build a network for payer contracts; commonly featuring joint governance between hospital and physician leadership, varying degree of MSO support and centralization, lackluster attraction for covered lives, little meaningful physician practice behavior modification, and little long-term loyalties from providers; *see also MSO, and PHO*

operational qualified HMO—an HMO that HCFA has determined provides basic and supplemental health services to all of its enrollees, and is organized and operated in accordance with applicable CFR-42, sections 417.168 and 417.169

OPHCOO—Office of Prepaid Health Care Operations and Oversight; once a part of the Public Health Service. This is the federal agency that oversees federal qualification and compliance for HMOs and eligibility for CMPs; previous names include the Health Maintenance Organization Service, the Office of Health Maintenance Organizations, and the Office of Prepaid Health Care

OPL—other party liability; language used within a COB statement

OPM—Office of Personnel Management; the federal agency that administers the FEHBP

optional renewable policy—health insurance contract that the insurer has the right to terminate at any policy anniversary, or, in some cases, at any premium date; on this date the insurer may add coverage limitations or increase premium rates

optometric service plan—a form of prepaid group vision care program; *see also vision carve out*

OR—operating room

organized delivery system—*see ODS*

orientation—*see new member orientation*

OSHA—Occupational Safety and Health Administration; a federal agency that regulates and investigates safety and health standards of jobs

OTC—over-the-counter drug; a pharmaceutical that may be sold without federal or state prescription requirements, and may be purchased without a doctor's order; a benefit option in many plans

other diagnoses—all conditions that exist at the time of admission or develop subsequently that affect the treatment received and/or length of stay, except diagnoses that relate to an earlier episode that have no bearing on the present hospital stay

other health insurance—*see OHI*

other party liability—includes programs to recover health care payment from other sources that are determined to have the first responsibility to pay, such as coordination of benefits (COB), third party liability, and Worker's Compensation; an insurer will seek the appropriate source of payment as part of the adjudication process, or pay the claim if no other party is liable; *see also COB, third-party liability, and worker's compensation*

outcome—also called health outcome, or the result of a process of prevention, detection, or treatment; an indicator of the effectiveness of health care measures upon patients; *see also outcomes measurement*

outcomes management—*see outcomes measurement*

outcomes measurement—a method of systematically monitoring a patient's medical or surgical intervention or nonintervention together with the associated responses, including measure of morbidity and functional status; findings from outcomes studies enable managed care entities to outline protocols according to their findings; *see also outcome*

outlier—within the context of statistical measurement of patient-related data, a patient that does not fall within a normal bell curve distribution of two or three standard deviations (depending on the selected statistical controls), such as a high utilizer of medical services, or longer ALOS

out-of-area—*see OOA*

out-of-area benefit—a covered benefit of health care insurance that specifically includes care that may be necessary while the member is out of the specified geographical area, or normal service area as outlined within the insurance plan

out-of-area coverage—*see out-of-area benefit*

out-of-area emergency—due to accidental bodily injury or other emergency medical condition, a member receives immediate medical treatment or services in a location other than the service area of the plan; in such an event, the plan will make the appropriate arrangements for the member's earliest possible discharge or transfer to an "in service area" participating provider

out-of-area transfer agreement—an agreement that permits a Blue Shield Plan subscriber who is moving to another geographical area to transfer from one participating plan to another

out-of-network—may consist of hospital care or other provider services that are rendered by nonparticipating provider entities, due to the purposeful selection by the enrollee or the

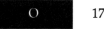

occurrence of an illness or injury while on out-of-area travel; some plans call for the member to pay the fees, while others allow for coverage under a higher copay by the member; *see also out-of-area, and out-of-plan referral*

out-of-plan referral—referrals to specialists who are not participating providers, which must be preauthorized by the system or plan medical director

out-of-pocket costs—*see OOP*

out-of-pocket limit—a stated limitation of out-of-pocket costs, which provides a comfort or guarantee to the patient that all costs will be provided, once the limit is reached for health services received during the contract year for all care except that which is outlined as excluded for coverage; *see also catastrophic insurance*

outpatient—an enrollee who receives treatment or services that do not consist of a inpatient admission to a hospital

outpatient drugs—a common additional benefit to members of HMOs; *see also additional benefits to Medicare risk*

over-the-counter drug—*see OTC*

P&T committee—pharmacy and therapeutics committee; a group that recommends the safe and effective use of prescriptions, and administers a standard drug formulary, generally consisting of providers from various specialties with common membership also representing pharmacy or resources functions within a medical group, hospital, health system, or health plan; *see also formulary*

PAC—preadmission certification; a certification that acute hospitalization or surgery is necessary, performed before the patient's admission; based on the judgment of medically appropriate care by a qualified peer

PACE—programs of all inclusive care for the elderly; in Medicaid parlance

package(d) pricing—a reimbursement strategy between providers and purchasers of health care that involves the offer of flat or fixed fees for all aspects of an episode of care, normally on a limited number of case types, which may include category-based pricing; the goal is to offer employers and insurers preferred pricing on DRGs that the provider can manage well due to improved care coordination, without setting a fixed fee for all diagnoses (or global); some episode pricing, such as $1,400 for a normal vaginal delivery, include a stated amount of prenatal (preadmission) and postnatal (postadmission) care, in addition to the delivery (DRG); best used with a large number of covered lives in order to spread risk; *see also DRG-specific per-case pricing, and global fee*

paid amount—the portion of a claim that is actually paid, consisting of the patient's payment, which may include copayment and the responsibility for balance billing, and third-party payment; *see also balance billing*

paid claims—the payment amount to providers to meet the terms of the contract by the health plan, excluding the enrolled member's responsibilities for out-of-pocket costs; *see also DFFS, FFS, global capitation, and out-of-pocket costs*

paid claims loss ratio—the amount of all paid claims, not including IBNR, divided by the revenue from all health plan premiums

paperless medical record—*see EMR*

PAR—Participating Physician and Supplier Program; any physician or supplier that agrees to accept assignment for the Medicare allowable payments for one year, who in turn receives fiscal and administrative incentives

par provider—short for participating provider; *see participating provider*

paramedical personnel—*see midlevel practitioner*

Part A—*see Medicare Part A*

Part B—*see Medicare Part B*

partial capitation—a capitation model or contract that involves a capitated payment (usually at a lower amount) plus a payment that is related to the actual cost of care and services; sometimes used as a method of slowly evolving toward the total capitation of providers within a medical group or market area; *see also capitation*

partial disability—inability to perform one or more functions of one's regular job; a key classification for disability plans or other coverage

partial hospitalization services—an appropriate, yet reduced-cost patient care setting for treatment or follow-up of mental health or substance abuse

partial risk contract—*see partial risk model*

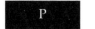

partial risk model—an agreement between an insured and insurer that transfers partial but not total risk; may involve a shared risk and payment arrangement between a plan and HCFA, where the FFS payments above or below a target capitation rate (i.e., 95% of the AAPCC) are shared between the plan and HCFA; variant models may include a corridor with an optional initial band with no cost sharing, a band with percentage cost sharing, and if necessary, an outer band in which FFS is paid, i.e., no gain or risk to the plan

participating hospital—a hospital that contracts to be a part of a network, system, or other managed care agreement, serving as a participating provider; *see also participating provider*

participating physician—a physician who contracts to be a part of a network, IPA, PPO, or other managed care entity, serving as a participating provider; *see also participating provider*

Participating Physician and Supplier Program—*see PAR*

participating provider—an individual provider, hospital, integrated delivery network, pharmacist, dentist, optometrist, chiropractor, podiatrist, nurse, group practice, nursing home, behavioral or mental health entity, skilled nursing facility, long-term care facility, or other medical institution agreeing to provide care or services to enrolled members of a particular plan, according to stated rates and conditions; in most prepayment relationships, including CHAMPUS and Medicare, the participating provider receives payment directly from the plan, but the patient must pay any cost share or deductible

participation—used to define the general level to which employees are willing to enroll for medical coverage (such as 50% participation of eligible employees who enroll for coverage, including eligible dependents); *see also market share, and penetration rate*

participation criteria—a written set of rules for initial acceptance or continued participation in a network, or other form of managed care entity; typically includes obligations of the provider as well as the entity, for compensation agreement, statements of liability limitations, terms for renewal or termination of the provider, and any agreements for claims submission, UR/QA, and patient referrals

partnership capitation model—a capitated arrangement in which a hospital and physician group jointly accept risk in a contract with an insurer; the hospital(s) and physician group(s) may create this arrangement in the absence of an MSO or PHO, or the partnership may be synonymous with an MSO or PHO; provides a faster alternative to gaining access to covered lives versus waiting until a comprehensive network is fully completed; *see also loyal physician contract strategy, MSO, and PHO*

partnership program—the CHAMPUS program that allows eligible beneficiaries to receive health care from civilian-sector providers who have been specifically approved to practice within the MTF, or to receive health care from military providers within civilian facilities; this program will be phased out and replaced by Resource Sharing under TRICARE; *see also CHAMPUS, Resource Sharing, and TRICARE*

party in interest—any director, officer, partner, or employee responsible for management or administration of an HMO; any person who is directly or indirectly the beneficial owner of more than 5% of the HMO equity; any person who is the beneficial owner of a mortgage, deed of trust, note, or other interest secured by, and valuing more than 5% of HMO assets; and for nonprofit HMO corporations, an incorporator or member of the corporation under applicable state corporation law

patient advocate—a representative within a hospital or health system who serves as the patient's liaison in order to ensure the receipt of adequate treatment, referral, proper charges, or to resolve other needs or concerns

patient broker—an intermediary agent who most often contracts with insurers, providers, and sometime medical groups, to recruit patients and increase managed care enrollment, either directly or through their employers; brokers receive a percent-

age of the annual premium for their service, which is normally less than the hiring entity would spend on marketing—hence the niche need that is filled by brokers; brokers are expected to focus on small business enrollment in upcoming years, particularly states with small business insurance reform; brokers assist employees with primary care physician selection, and serve as ongoing member services, assuming they are paid beyond the initial recruitment; *see also patient broker channeling incentive*

patient broker channeling incentive—the action by patient brokers to direct or channel patients to a particular source of care or health plan enrollment, as a result of being financially rewarded, through either a salary structure, bonus, or commission; *see also channeling, patient broker, and physician channeling incentive*

patient care redesign—*see patient care reengineering, and QI*

patient care reengineering—"clean sheet of paper" approach of bringing positive change to health care in an attempt to cut costs while maintaining quality; in accordance with the overall theory of reengineering, which allows the team to design a preferred process as if no process were already in place; this method searches for a more appropriate use of health care resources, both within the traditional hospital and outpatient settings, and across the continuum of care, and includes the other disciplines of UR, case management, and discharge planning; advocates suggest reengineering as the primary way to cut costs, while others emphasize cutting procedures; *see also QI*

patient dumping—the practice of refusing services to uninsured indigent patients or transferring them to a public hospital or a private, nonprofit hospital willing to treat indigents

patient incentive—contemporary managed care strategies include ways to give incentives to patients, since they control significant ability to contain costs based on selection decisions and other behavior; some plans allow for reduced premium with evidence of frequent exercise or other risk-aversive behavior such as not smoking; other plans reduce or eliminate copay for patients who choose low-cost physicians and hospitals—a strategy that is strengthened by offering patients a guide of local cost comparisons; some providers include contract mandates for payers to send cost comparisons to patients, knowing that their facility is a low-cost leader; *see also physician channeling incentive*

patient protection act—*see PPA*

patient recruiter—*see patient broker*

patient relations representative—*see member services*

patient retention—the success of a medical group, patient broker, provider, or health plan in retaining enrolled patient-members, from one contract period to the next; often rewarded with a percentage bonus pay structure for member services, or as a primary pay component of brokers; high retention rates result from effective communication and service quality, quick response to questions, hassle-free policies, fast payment, and most importantly, satisfaction with the PCP; patient disenrollment surveys aid member services staff in retention; retention is critical to reducing administrative costs, due to the high cost of recruiting and educating new members, particularly in Medicare or Medicaid; *see also patient broker, patient retention bonus program, and physician patient retention program*

patient retention bonus program—a program that is created as an incentive for member services representative to provide excellent service to support enrolled members; normally operate on a percentage measure of existing members retained, with a bonus payment added to the base salary when a goal is met, or with added bonus payment on a sliding scale for enhanced retention; *see also new member orientation*

patient satisfaction—a critical element toward understanding what issues cause a patient to select a particular health care system, and what issues are most likely to influence changing their current care affiliation, for either the physician, the hospital, or the health plan; required as an essential component of various accreditation reviews and a growing set of employer standards; the responsive use of survey data can assist increased market penetration and enhance health care quality; involves survey and questionnaire theory and application, automation and other techniques to make customer participation easy, and language translation for multicultural markets

patient telemanagement—the periodic follow-up of a patient by telephone; the goal is to avoid an undetected or uncommunicated patient need, which may become aggravated to the point of requiring more expensive intervention, or an office visit; may be performed by various skill levels, depending upon the patient need: physician, nurse, technician, or even a volunteer; often telemanagement involves questions to chronically ill or elderly patients that help to ensure compliance in taking medication properly, or to detect weight gain or loss; remarkable savings have resulted from telemanagement

pay or play—a strategy to bring insurance to individuals, through either federal or state laws; a federal proposal was drafted but not implemented to require employers either to provide health insurance for their workers or to pay a tax that would enable the government to provide insurance; variations of the federal proposal include a national spending increase ceiling tied to GNP by the year 2000, a national commission to negotiate fees with providers, individual cost share, and income surtax; New Jersey levied a charge on insurers that did not participate in their pay or play plan (called Individual Health Coverage), to cover losses of insurers who play; *see also universal access*

payer—also called payor and carrier; *see carrier*

payment level—the amount paid for each provider unit of service, consisting of the amount paid by the insured and the insurer; the capitated payments to providers, or insurers; *see also allowable charge*

payment rate—*see payment level*

payroll deduction—each employing entity that provides payroll deductions as a means of paying employees' contributions for health benefits or provides a health benefits plan that does not require an employee contribution must, with the consent of an employee who selects the HMO option, arrange for the employee's contribution, if any, to be paid through payroll deductions

PBM—pharmacy benefit management; a relatively young industry that specializes in reducing the amount of cost for pharmaceuticals, either in support of an HMO or a hospital-based system; PBMs now connect most of the U.S. pharmacies via computer network with programs to provide data reporting, educational information directed toward least-cost prescribing alternatives, software to support drug-to-drug interactions within an entire community and to keep patients from receiving redundant and costly services; some PBMs are independent organizations, while others are subsidiaries of drug companies or insurance companies; PBMs can reduce the amount of monthly PMPM cost of pharmacy services, from an approximate savings range of $1-$3 PMPM relative to an overall pharmacy cost of $9-$13 for a commercial population, not including Medicare or Medicaid

PCCM—primary care case management; a more specialized definition of case management, found in Medicaid programs and other settings that require a gatekeeper to coordinate and manage primary care services, referrals, pre-admission certification, and other medical or rehabilitative services; the primary advantage of PCCM for Medicaid eligibles has been to provide increased access to PCP while reducing use of hospital outpatient departments and emergency rooms; encouraged within Medicare Choices to provide PCP coordination for patients being treated by a wide variety of specialists but who no longer have a PCP for oversight; *see also gatekeeper model, and PCP*

PCCO—physician-sponsored coordinated care organization; a term used by the AMA and others to describe a proposed managed care entity that could enter into direct relationships with

HCFA to provide Medicare risk care, like a self-insured plan, because it pays out its own benefits using its own resources and assets in conjunction with reinsurance as a guarantee against excess claims; a PCCO would not, as proposed, be required to comply with insurance regulation; PCCOs would differ from PSNs, in that they are physician, and not hospital-provider sponsored—with the goal of higher quality through physician decision making, with lower cost by eliminating the insurer

PCM—primary care manager; *see PCP*

PCN—primary care network; a group of primary care physicians who have joined together to share the risk of providing care to their patients who are members of a given health plan; the basic formation of a PCP is to support care coverage for a plan within a contract, or region within a contract; some contracts outline minimum requirements for the network either in terms of PCPs/1,000 patients, or total PCPs within a region as out-lined in the contract

PCP—primary care provider or primary care physician; a physi-cian, the majority of whose practice is devoted to internal med-icine, family/general practice and pediatrics; an OB/Gyn may be considered a primary care physician, and some networks provide a focused retraining for OB/Gyns so that they may enter into risk contracts for a population of women patients; *see also gatekeeper model*

PCP capitation—the portion of the capitation that is entirely directed toward payment for primary care services, i.e., is paid to the primary care provider

PCP quota law—a growing debate is taking place within state legislative agendas to set a minimum restriction on the percent-age of primary care physicians that must graduate from medi-cal schools, so that a sufficient number of PCPs are produced for the changing health care market needs; six states have laws and others are considering limits—Arizona, Minnesota, North Carolina, Tennessee, Washington, and Wisconsin

PCR—physician contingency reserve; one term among a multitude of applications using a set-aside to guard against future medical claims expenses, in the hopes that the money will not be needed and can be paid out according to an agreement; normally a higher percentage is kept in reserves if the physicians do not have a lot of successful experience in managing care within expenses; assuming that providers succeed in managing care properly, there is reward for taking risk as evidenced by the payout of the reserves; also called risks pool, withhold pool, bonus pool, capitation pool; *see also capitation, and physician production formula*

PEC—preexisting condition; any single or multiple physical and/or mental impairment or disease of an enrollee that exists before the insurance begins; many plans have a range of the time period, before which an enrollee can begin to receive care for preexisting conditions, to establish the fact that their health condition is relatively stable, such as for posttransplant enrollees; the lack of mandate for insurers to cover preexisting conditions is a volatile legislative topic at state and federal levels

pediatric hotline or triage system—one type of specialized telephone triage system for pediatric application; pediatric practices may choose to install a telephone system to either reduce the evening and weekend call demands for their practice, or to reduce unnecessary office visits; some practices that have only a small portion of their revenue derived from capitation have actually seen office visits fall to the point where there is negatively impacted revenue beyond a desired outcome; *see also telephone triage system*

peer pregnancy counselor—the selection and education of counselors from low-income neighborhoods, who serve as peers for pregnant women; a valuable strategy toward improving health outcomes for low birthweight and other issues as a result of deliveries by young, low income women; Medicaid tests within Aid to Dependent Children (ADC), General Assistance (GA), and other applications have yielded remarkable results, particularly with women who have higher social illness, substance abuse, or other medical problems; expanded use is growing in a number of urban areas

peer review—an evaluation usually performed within the boundaries of the same geographical area and medical specialty, by reviewing a patient's case using a group of unbiased practicing physicians to judge the effectiveness and efficiency of care rendered, responsible for review against the overutilization or misuse of a plan's benefits; *see also PRO*

peer review group—a peer review entity that normally serves within a medical group, hospital, local health system, or community, versus the function served by a PRO to review care, resolve appeals, or ensure ethics in medical practice; *see also peer review, and PRO*

peer review organization—*see PRO*

penetration rate—the rate at which eligible enrollees decide to become covered in a managed care plan; if an HMO enrolls 2,000 out of 20,000 eligible patients, the penetration rate is 10%

per case—*see case rate*

per contract per month—the amount of capitated health care resources or the health insurance premium for each contract holder, or member, each month; *see PMPM*

per diem or per diem reimbursement—a reimbursement mechanism that pays a provider (normally an acute care facility) an established or negotiated rate per day rather than reimburse all hospital charges as billed; although many providers seek to transfer the reward for taking risk from the HMO (and getting a global capitation), most plans currently reimburse provider systems or hospitals on a per diem basis; per diems may be established for major categories of care, such as medical/surgical, obstetrics, mental health, ICU, oncology, cardiac, or minimum use per service; may include elements for incremental sliding scale volume, ancillary services used, contribution margin, mix of days by type, or ALOS; *see also prospective per diem*

per member per month—*see PMPM*

per member per year—*see PMPY*

per subscriber per month—the amount of capitated health care resources or the health insurance premium for each subscribing patient, or member, each month; *see PMPM*

per thousand members per year—*see PTMPY*

percent of premium—the percent of any element measured against the price of the monthly premium that an HMO charges for a particular benefit plan; so, if an HMO charges $100 per month to the patient, with various PMPM amounts expended on delivery systems, hospitals, PCPs, administration, specialists, drugs, risk management, profit, and other elements, then a profit of $5 is 5% of premium; considered to be the greatest financial risk for reimbursement arrangements based on a percent of premium (versus a less risky continuum ranging from billed charges, DFFS, per diem, case rate, and PMPM)

performance-based channeling—*see channeling*

performance-based physician pay—any of multiple methods to reimburse physicians by providing bonus or incentive pay for a certain type of utilization or performance behavior, ranging from salary to full personal capitation; *see also DFFS, FFS, full personal capitation, physician production formula, physician salary plus bonus*

performance measure—*see metric*

performance measures—a system that aids providers or insurers in making decisions about health care or to enhance health status and the quality of patient outcomes; the Joint Commission has outlined a health care network performance matrix to include clinical performance, health status, satisfaction of patients, practitioners, and purchasers, process effectiveness, and the communication and education of patients, providers, and the public

performance standard—the specified minimum threshold that a provider must maintain according to an agreement, which may include measurements regarding the quality of care, timeliness of patient access or medical record completion, workload volume, or office hours; the agreement may further outline the bonus or penalty structures that become activated, depending on actual performance

periodic interim payment—*see PIP*

personal capitation—*see full personal capitation*

personal injury—*see injury*

personal letter—a common practice of medical groups, providers, or insurers, either as a part of direct mail marketing strategy, or to create another type of influence upon patients, such as to make them aware of a provider's new affiliation with an insurer that can lower their cost of health care, to inform them of the list of all insurers with which the provider is affiliated, or to gain their support on behalf of a local hospital or medical group that is about to be excluded by a payer; personal letters from physicians can be more effective than those from insurers in gaining the patient's attention; *see also direct mail*

phantom billing—billing for services not performed; *see also coding creep*

phantom or ghost population—enrollees who do not have a defined actuarial experience in terms of their use of health care resources, but will likely begin to use medical resources under a proposed contract

pharmacy and therapeutics committee—*see P&T committee*

pharmacy benefit management—*see PBM*

pharmacy carve out—within a capitation environment, pharmacy supplies and services are often provided through a carve out from the PMPM or pricing structure for a specified range of coverage; the most competitive regional pharmacy subcontractors, or national pharmacy benefit managers, are capable of delivering these requirements at a savings of $1-3 PMPM relative to an overall pharmacy cost of $9-13 PMPM for a commercial population; *see also PBM*

PHCO—physician–hospital–community organization; may be compared to a physician–hospital organization, with the addition of community governance representation

PHO—physician–hospital organization; an IPA associated with a hospital, often initiated by the hospital that provides management services; features a contracting mechanism for obtaining "covered lives," generally with 50:50 physician and hospital control and hospital financed; the benefits allow physicians to retain autonomy, and aid progress toward full integration or capitation, while the limitations include strained relationships with independent physicians, and possible difficulties over utilization control, division of revenue, and panel selection; only half of the states require license of PHOs that assume only partial risk

PHS—public health service; often used in reference to the PHS Act, paragraph 1310(d), which defines qualification requirements for an HMO to be approved by HCFA

physician behavior-retention incentives—since the leading reason for member disenrollment is dissatisfaction with the primary care physician, some medical groups, providers, and health plans have implemented strong ties between physician behavior (complaints and problems that lead to the patient's selection of another physician) and physician pay incentives; problematic behavior is particularly costly for the more sizable monthly Medicare risk revenue—and failure to link behavior to pay could cause continued physician reward with simultaneous losses for the medical group, provider, or plan

physician channeling—the ability and result of physician influence upon patients to redirect their decision to choose either a health plan or a hospital, based upon input from the physician, since the average patient's ties to the physician are stronger than to the plan or the hospital; physicians will channel toward a new HMO, if the current HMO (of the patient's enrollment and physician's affiliation) does not suit the physician, for reasons of policy, payment, or service, the physician notifies the patient of the intent to cut HMO ties, in hopes that the patient will follow to another HMO; similarly with a hospital, the physician may encourage the patient to seek upcoming hospital care at a specific hospital based upon its physician service accommodation, exclusive hospital contract relationships, or preferred payment or bonus sharing; *see also Medicare marketing–physician steering, physician referral service, and specialist channeling*

physician channeling incentive—incentive pay to physicians from insurers, based on their success in channeling workload to low-cost providers; insurer contracts with providers often contain a sliding scale structure for added volume to the hospital, and increased hospital discounts to the payer, in response to channeling by physicians, increased market penetration for providers, and savings to the insurer

physician contingency reserve—*see PCR*

physician exchange, guide, hotline, matching, or exchange—*see physician referral service; see also physician on-line directory*

physician–hospital organization—*see PHO*

physician mix—a description of comparison between the number or percentage of PCPs versus specialists in a group, IPA, IDN, or HMO; early managed care markets may be in the range of 35% PCPs/65% specialists, while more mature markets are 50%/50% or greater, in recognition of PCPs as a key to managing cost; *see also full personal capitation*

physician on-line directory—a type of physician referral service that can be accessed from a computer, through a variety of on-line services; on-line directories can provide printable details of the physician's services, medical capabilities, office address and map of the location, and patient access information; most on-line directories provide one-way information to the patient, but some provide interactive two-communication features; directories may be sponsored by any medical group, provider, or health plan wishing to add this recruitment service; *see also physician channeling, and physician referral service*

physician patient retention program—any program that obtains patient data regarding their relative satisfaction and retention statistics, and then makes some decision that links the physician's role or behavior in retaining patients, and decisions involving the physician's continued employment, promotion, salary, or bonus pay; various programs have evolved out of recognition of the physician's central role in retention, giving increased value to physician service quality as a component of rated performance

Physician Payment Review Commission—*see PPRC*

physician peer pressure—used to describe any type of strategy that is directed toward making the practice of medicine more efficient, or obtaining improved patient outcomes; such as the presentation of utilization data that compares physicians within a panel or pod-level risk group, continued physician education, peer review, or the actual creation of physician pods; *see also peer review, and pod-level risk pool*

physician practice management—*see MSO*

physician production formula—when capitated care is provided by a group of physicians, versus capitation at the personal physician-level, a common payment mechanism involves a distribution of funds to physicians based on the fee-for-service care that each physician has provided during the period; this method rewards a higher number of visits or procedures with a higher payment; *see also full personal capitation, and PCR*

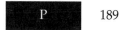

physician redirecting—*see physician channeling; see also Medicare marketing–physician steering*

physician referral service—a "yellow pages" written directory service, or a telephonic service that assists patients in selecting a physician, based on the needs of the patient; a goal of the service is to recruit patients to a medical group, hospital, or health plan that pays for the referral service—or to convert patients from existing relationships with another medical group, hospital, or health plan; often the sponsor of the physician referral service is masked, to minimize the appearance of steering patients; if a provider or medical group does not receive the coverage desired from an insurer, it can create its own service; also called physician hotlines, doctors referral line, or physician exchange or guide; *see also physician on-line directory*

physician salary plus bonus—a physician payment method that involves a specified salary plus the physician contingency reserve bonus; the bonus is structured to incentivize desired provider behavior, which may range from patient satisfaction to low utilization of downstream services; *see also downstream costs, PCR, and physician production formula*

physician service quality—those aspects of a physician's manner, conduct, or behavior in providing patient care that are not related to the quality of care or medical decisions; examples include either the presence or absence of patient complaints, problems of untimely patient access (which may indicate the physician has enrolled too many patients, or other problems with practice efficiency), indications of a caring or compassionate attitude, ability to answer patient questions, or other factors within the physician's control; low physician service quality leads to patient disenrollment or even malpractice claims, which may or may not impact physician pay, depending on the use of a physician patient retention program; *see also physician patient retention program*

physician services—services that are either personally furnished for an individual patient by a physician, or contributing to the diagnosis or treatment of the individual patient; ordinarily required to be performed by a physician; or in the case of anesthesiology, radiology, or laboratory services, additional special regulatory requirements (stated in regulations 42 CFR 405.552/.554/.556 for each of these specialty areas) are met; the importance of "physician services" classification comes from an October 1983 policy, which stated that only inpatient services not covered under Part A of the prospective payment system for hospitals will be physician services, except for direct medical education and capital costs—as a result, physician services are paid on the basis of reasonable charges

physician-sponsored coordinated care organization—*see PCCO*

physician unit cost hospital pool—a risk sharing strategy between a hospital and an affiliated medical group that provides an incentive for the physicians to assist the hospital in lowering daily inpatient unit costs (understanding that physicians control about two-thirds of inpatient costs); structured somewhat like the hospital standard risk pool, allowing hospitals to charge the pool as each inpatient day is provided for patients, based on the existing full per diem rate (not on estimated cost per case, fixed costs, or incremental costs as in other cost pools); end-of-year calculations determine what savings may be shared with physicians, and next year's unit per diem costs are lowered according to current year's actual costs; *see also hospital DRG risk pool, hospital standard risk pool, hospital variable cost risk pool, and provider inpatient cost control*

physician work—the specific measurement of physician time, effort, skill, judgment, and stress from risk that is associated with the Medicare relative value scale; *see also RVS*

Physician's Current Procedural Terminology—*see CPT*

pie meeting—*see Medicare marketing–social recruitment*

PIP—periodic interim payment; an advance payment transaction from a payer to a provider that represents some portion of the lag factor for services rendered within an IBNR context; the recent trend is for payers to decrease or eliminate PIPs, based

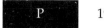

on their clout, which impacts the provider's financial statements in many ways, such as increased accounts receivable; *see also IBNR, and lag factor*

place of service—now that an expanded continuum of care is available to the patient, the location where health services are rendered (acute hospital, LTC center, doctor's office, or home) becomes an important consideration, for actual treatment and for reporting purposes

PLI—professional liability insurance; *see malpractice insurance*

PMC—physician management corporation; *see MSO*

PMPM—per member per month; the revenue or cost of a risk payment that is typically made to providers by HMOs, for providing a defined amount of care for each enrolled patient each month

PMPY—per member per year; same as PMPM but for a year

pod-level risk pool or pod—a group/pod of 5 to 15 primary care physicians (many prefer 4–6) given a collective risk pool based upon a budget for a distinct population assigned to the pod; physicians earn money back from the physician contingency reserve or risk pool by reducing hospital and other "downstream" costs; pods are more effective with clinical protocols, advanced sharing of information (both in the didactic and automated sense), and peer pressure, which could be full personal capitation; some pods include specialists, physician leaders, and partial administrator monitoring or assistance; *see also downstream costs, and full personal capitation*

point of attachment—within the context of stop loss insurance, the point of attachment is the level over which the insurance begins to cover added claims loss; so an HMO, hospital network, or medical practice might purchase stop loss insurance with an attachment at $50,000, over which amount the insurance covers the loss; *see also stop loss*

point of care—used to describe computer technology that provides capability at the point of care to support order entry, file retrieval, computerized patient record completion or access; point of care systems eliminate double data entry, reduce delay, and add to the efficiency of clinicians

point of service—*see POS plan*

point of total government responsibility—*see POTGR*

policy holder—*see insured*

political subdivision—within the context of public entities that are employing units for employee health benefit plans under federally qualified HMOs, a political subdivision includes: counties, parishes, townships, cities, municipalities, towns, villages, and incorporated villages

pool (risk pool)—a portion of payments for services rendered is placed within a pool as a source for any subsequent claims that exceed projections, for a defined group of patients or product that is defined by size, or geographic location; funds that remain in the pool after a specified term are paid out to providers, thereby creating an incentive for lower utilization; the potential for "up-side" payout from risk pools is the basis for providers to convert to a managed care style of practice versus FFS, because although the reimbursements are compressed as managed care becomes more mature within the region, the provider is capable of seeing larger populations of patients for less cost per patient

pooling—aggregating the risk for a number of groups into a single pool

portability—a desirable feature that allows health coverage to be extended after small business employees either lose a job or are transferred from one location to another, versus losing coverage; an alternate definition within state laws allows employees that are changing jobs to have the waiting period or underwriting requirements at their new location to be reduced because of

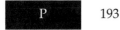

previous enrollment; *see also group-to-group portability, group-to-individual portability, and Kassebaum-Kennedy Health Coverage Bill*

POS mandate—*see mandatory point-of-service*

POS plan—point of service; this plan provides an either/or flexibility for an enrollee to choose to receive a service from a participating provider (managed care, with no or low deductibles/copays) or nonparticipating provider (FFS, with higher deductibles/copays), with corresponding benefit or "penalty" of copay depending upon the level of benefit selected, which is designed to encourage use of network providers; POS maintains the popularity of choice by offering the typical HMO provision, PPO, fee-for-service indemnity, or combinations of each; in many POS plans, enrollees coordinate their care needs through the PCP; HMOs pay nonparticipating providers at an FFS rate; also called HMO swing-out plan or out-of-plan rider to an HMO; *see also HMO, out-of-network, and PPO*

postacute care—one of many types of health care settings after the traditional acute care, or as an alternative to acute hospitalization, along the continuum of care, including: long-term, skilled-nursing care, home care, hospice, rehabilitation, and outpatient surgery; this segment of care has enjoyed increased utilization because of its lower cost to acute care, but may be in for reductions in Medicare and Medicaid reimbursement, depending on legislation; *see also aftercare, and continuum of care*

postdischarge case management—a function that features a case manager who specializes in the management of high-risk and chronic care patients, by providing any necessary home health arrangements, follow-up telephone contact to assess patient status and need for further visits, medication assessment, and compliance review; *see also case manager, chronic disease center, and CM*

post-site visit analysis—the third step of HCFA's procedures to federally qualify an HMO or CMP, involving submission of a written report from each HCFA reviewer to the Qualification or

Eligibility Officer, followed by a report of recommendation by that officer to the senior staff

POTGR—point of total government responsibility; in the current TRICARE managed care support contracts, the risk corridor on the downside of loss calls for Tier 1 of contractor responsibility to be borne up to 101%, Tier 2 shared at 80% for government, and 20% for the HMO, until the POTGR is reached in which the contractor has absorbed losses equal to the cumulative profit for all option periods completed (plus an additional contractor-proposed amount of equity, at a minimum of $15 million/year). After the POTGR is reached, the government absorbs all losses; *see also TRICARE*

PPA—patient protection act; the name given to legislation introduced in many state capitals since 1995; proposals often contain any willing provider provisions (to allow any willing provider to join a panel versus allowing physician deselection by the insurer) or other standards aimed at protecting the provider, such as requirements for disclosure or continuity of care by the insurer; Maryland and Oregon enacted PPA legislation in 1995, with over 20 other states considering bills; *see also antimanaged care legislation, AWP, and exclusivity*

PPA—preferred provider arrangement; an arrangement made by an employer with providers to provide a loosely organized model of care, similar to the PPO

PPGP—prepaid group practice; emphasis on the practice, and not the health plan; a formal association of three or more physicians that provides a defined set of services to persons over a specified time period in return for a fixed periodic prepayment made in advance for the use of service

PPN—preferred provider network; any number or mix of providers that form a network for managed care contracting with a health plan, or hospital entity; used to describe the participating providers of the Department of Defense TRICARE insurer (managed care support contractor)

PPO—preferred provider organization; may be the description of a plan or an affiliation of providers seeking contracts with a plan by virtue of their ability to cover a broad geographical area, or provide multispecialty skills; incentives for providers to participate include quick turnaround of claims payment, a valuable pool of patients, most often FFS or DFFS payment; payer incentive is negotiated discounts to FFS; a physician-sponsored PPO increasingly will bear risk when seeking arrangement with insurance companies or self-insured companies; there is great consensus that PPOs are early stage managed care relationships that are formed in response to HMO pressure or competition, but do not bring the same savings as HMOs; *see also DFFS, FFS, and HMO*

PPRC—physician payment review commission; beginning in 1986, this group was created by Congress through the 1985 COBRA to establish a process for determining a relative value scale for payment of physician services, to comment on the HHS proposal to establish a process for determining the inherent reasonableness of payment for certain services, and to prepare an annual report to Congress; under the most recent Democratic administration proposal for Medicare, the PPRC (which primarily sets Part B fees) is retained, together with ProPAC (which primarily sets Part A fees); the failed Republican budget plan sought to combine PPRC with ProPAC, and another proposed House bill would have created a Medicare Payment Review Commission (MPRC); *see also ProPAC*

PPS—prospective payment system; for Medicare services as established by Title VI of the Social Security Amendments of 1983, developed and implemented by HCFA to pay health care facilities for Medicare patients; this system replaced the retrospective cost-based method that was begun in 1968; the primary prevention against premature discharge of patients is the presence of sound quality assurance programs; *see also prospective reimbursement*

practice expense—the portion of a physician's expenses that is related to the costs of running the office/practice, such as overhead, office equipment and supplies, salaries, benefits; all expenses of a nonphysician nature; one of the three components of the Medicare relative value scale; *see also RVS*

practice expense relative value—the average or relative amount of practice expense incurred for any medical service, measured in units per service that are used within the Medicare relative value scale; *see also RVS*

practice guideline—*see medical protocols*

practice parameter—*see medical protocols*

practitioner—*see provider*

preadmission certification or review—*see PAC*

preadmission education—education for the patient and/or family members before the time of admission, in order to provide information about the likely events following admission, treatment alternatives, rehabilitation and recovery expectations, and the anticipated flow within the hospital from admission to discharge; the goal of preadmission education is to make the patient and/or family aware of the hospitalization process, to reduce surprise and confusion later, which may assist reducing LOS; *see also discharge planning*

preadmission testing—X-ray and laboratory testing performed in a hospital's outpatient department before admission for nonemergency surgery or other medical treatment; for insurance purposes, these tests will be covered under hospital inpatient benefits if they are part of hospital admission procedures

preauthorization—payment for most services provided to a beneficiary of a managed care contract will be made only after someone in the managed care company agrees that the treatment is needed and sanctions it

precertification—*see PAC*

preexisting condition—*see PEC*

preexisting condition exclusion—*see preexisting condition limits*

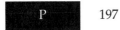

preexisting condition limits—a growing number of states have passed laws that establish a maximum waiting period during which insurers can deny health coverage to a member with preexisting conditions, such as 6 or 12 months

preferred provider—any entity defined as a provider who has agreed to contract for the provision of health services for all enrolled members of a plan; *see also participating provider, PPO, and provider*

preferred provider arrangement—same as a PPO, but sometimes used to refer to a looser arrangement between the payer and provider, in which the payer makes the arrangements rather than the provider

preferred provider network—*see PPN*

preferred provider organization—*see PPO*

premium—an amount of money that is paid to a health plan by a subscriber or an employer group in exchange for providing stated health care benefits (and claims processing, or various other administrative services, as specified); *see also contributory program, and noncontributory plan*

premium support system—a term used as the opposite of a service reimbursement system, to define a futuristic Medicare system that shifts emphasis to having the government pay a certain portion of an insurance policy premium for a beneficiary, rather than continuing in the tradition of reimbursing for a stated level of services

preoperational qualified HMO—an entity that HCFA has determined will, when it becomes operational, be a qualified HMO; within 30 days of HCFA's determination as preoperational, the HMO must provide assurance that it will become operational within 60 days, with the ability to meet all requirements of an operationally qualified HMO; *see also operational qualified HMO*

prepaid care—any health care plan offering potential patients an opportunity to pay for their health care needs on an installment basis prior to getting sick, similar to an insurance policy; the incentive for the patient is to receive care as needed for free or for a small copayment, the incentive for the health plan or HMO is to keep the difference between premium revenues and medical care and administrative costs

prepaid group practice—*see PPGP*

prepaid group practice plan—a plan providing care to a given population by PCPs accepting fixed periodic prepayments; *see also HMO, and PMPM*

prepaid health plan—contract between an insurer and a subscriber or group of subscribers whereby the plan provides a specified set of health benefits in return for a periodic premium; *see also HCPP*

prepaid program—*see prepaid health plan*

prescription drug—a medication that can only be sold by a pharmacy or dispensed after an order by an appropriately licensed physician; for medications approved by the FDA for sale under federal or state law

prevailing charge—the fee most frequently charged in an area by a group of physicians determines the prevailing charge; in the case of Medicare it could almost be defined as "the level of charge which is allowed to prevail," and the charge would cover 75% of the customary charges made for similar services in the same locality; this maximum Medicare rate is controlled by an economic index; other plans may pay a different percentage based on the prevailing charge; *see also reasonable and customary charge*

prevention measures—indicators of the frequency and effectiveness of the preventive care provided to the enrollee population

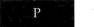

prevention protocols—a subset of medical protocols that focuses on preventing disease or the onset of other chronic conditions; prevention guidelines are the result from clinical studies and trials; an effective use of prevention protocols is to educate patients through a variety of individual or group settings, and distributing written material or patient self-help literature that will be available in time of need

preventive care—care and treatment that is given with the objective of precluding illness or hospitalization; a program that stresses education, early detection, and early treatment of conditions, generally including immunizations and routine physical examinations

price fixing—the conspiracy by two or more separate legal and economic entities to establish a market pricing mechanism; price fixing is overcome by formation of a single economic entity, since a single entity cannot conspire against itself

primary care—general medical care that is provided by family practitioners, pediatricians, general medical officers, internal medicine physicians, and sometimes includes care to women that is provided by OB/Gyn; *see also secondary care and tertiary care*

primary care capitation—a system of payment that provides a specified amount to each PCP for each enrolled member, i.e., PMPM; the amount is likely determined through the result of negotiation, but is based on the actuarial determination of primary care utilization costs for a comparable sample of patients; a portion of the capitation payment may be a withhold; some capitation experience shows that the preferred models evolve from initially having from 5 to 7 primary care physicians in a common risk- and profit-sharing group, also called a "pod," which is designed to help them learn the clinical practices best supporting managed care, with the ultimate model involving the personal capitation of PCPs, who are responsible for the "downstream" costs of specialist care and diagnostic procedures; *see also PMPM, pod-level risk pool, and withhold*

primary care case management—*see PCCM*

primary care network—*see PCN*

primary care pods—*see pod-level risk pool*

primary care physician—*see PCP*

primary care provider—*see PCP*

primary coverage—within the context of coordination of benefits, this term refers to the coverage plan that pays for eligible
expenses without recouping from another plan

principle of payment—the monthly advance payment equivalent to the HMO's or CMP's per capita rate of payment for each
beneficiary who is registered in HCFA records as a Medicare
enrollee; *see also adjustment to payment, and reduction of payments*

prior authorization—*see preadmission certification, and preauthorization*

private label HMO—an HMO that is formed through the lease of
an existing HMO license by a provider or PHO-type group that
includes physician investment, giving the health plan (which
likely has a low market penetration in the area) the advantage
of local market hospital brand name identification and loyalty,
by naming the plan after the hospital as a private label product;
a partnership between HMO and provider within a given market, which allows a division of responsibilities between partners (such as grievance service, marketing, premium collection,
responsibility for risk, and other responsibilities of an insurer)
according to a contract; sometimes referred to as the renting of
an HMO license by a provider; *see also HMO, ODS, PHO, PSN,
and retail HMO*

privileges—formal authority by an HMO or hospital-based system to treat patients at a hospital or within a system as granted
by a governing authority; *see also credentialing*

PRO—peer review organization or professional review organization; enacted under TEFRA in 1982 as a physician-sponsored entity responsible for the review of appropriateness and medical necessity of admissions, readmissions, and discharges for Medicare and Medicaid, quality of care, and the appropriateness of the medical setting when matched against professional criteria or standards; these entities must maintain and lower admission rates, and reduce ALOS while ensuring quality of care; Medicare PROs contract with HCFA; also called Professional Standards Review Organization (PSRO); *see also PSRO*

professional development—includes a spectrum of activities directed toward physician mentoring, training, or career enhancement; may consist of encouraging board certification, providing continuing medical education, offering tailored education in managed care to assist in cost-effective delivery, counseling on peer data or performance, encouragement to stay with the group or firm, and ultimate decisions for retention or separation

professional health care services—any professional health care services immediately incident to the care of patients including, but not limited to, the furnishing of food, beverages, medications, or appliances in connection with such services and the postmortem handling of human bodies

professional liability insurance—*see malpractice insurance*

professional review organization—*see PRO*

profile—health care data that are collected and reviewed to give insight into the utilization of services during various periods for a given population; a profile may be analyzed for an individual provider, a group practice, a health plan, or market area; *see also provider profiling*

profiling—*see profile*

ProPAC—Prospective Payment Assessment Commission; the group that advises Congress on Medicare payment issues (primarily Part A) and receives analytical support from 25 staff positions; *see also MPRC, and PPRC*

proration—a change of policy benefits that also may bring a change in premium, due to an enrolled member having other insurance or a change in job status

prospective payment—*see prospective reimbursement*

Prospective Payment Assessment Commission—*see ProPAC*

prospective payment system—*see PPS*

prospective per diem—*see per diem*

prospective pricing—setting a specific total, all-inclusive price for a service prior to delivery of the service, often on a DRG basis, usually established by the plan or payer and not by the provider, but may be the result of negotiation; *see also per diem*

prospective rate per case—*see case rate*

prospective rate per group—the hospital charges the HMO on the basis of the federally recognized diagnostic-related grouping (DRG) classification, which is widely used to reimburse hospitals for services to Medicare patients

prospective reimbursement—a prepayment plan for health care services that are to be provided according to contractual rates and terms during the stated period of agreement; this method involves establishing in advance the full amount of rates of payment that are acceptable, followed by the payment of these rates regardless of the actual experience or costs incurred; *see also experience rating, FFS, and global capitation*

prospective review—a function of utilization review that is directed toward establishing the medical necessity, appropriateness, and validity for reimbursement of care before an admission or provision of care; many health plans and providers adhere to listings of what services require a prospective review; *see also concurrent review, retrospective review, and UM*

provider—the generic term used to describe a physician, pharmacist, dentist, optometrist, chiropractor, podiatrist, nurse, hospital, group practice, nursing home, behavioral or mental health entity, skilled nursing facility, long-term care facility, pharmacy, other medical institution, or any individual or group of individuals that provides health care services; a distinction of the term provider, versus supplier, within Medicare policy, will determine payment on a charge basis for suppliers, but a prospective or retrospective cost-related basis for providers

provider arrangements—in the application process to HCFA to become a federally qualified HMO, there must be evidence of arrangements for basic health services in the requested area at the time the application is submitted, including either the explicit evidence of service to Medicare members or specific payment arrangements for services to Medicare members in provider contracts, or both; the application includes the listing of existing or draft contracts or letters of intent for staff (physicians, non-physicians, or non-staff physicians), group (member physicians, member non-physicians, non-member physicians, or non-member non-physicians), IPA (member physicians, member non-physicians, non-member physicians, non-member non-physicians), Direct Contract HMO physicians, laboratory services, X-ray services, hospitals, home health, and other services

provider audit—a review of the medical care delivered by a provider, in terms of medical record documentation, claim form, medical necessity, patient survey, and quality of care

provider broker—*see patient broker*

provider directory—*see physician referral service*

provider–employer risk pool—may be used in various direct contracting or care system models, to share year-end surplus or deficit between provider and coalition members, based on the difference between budgeted capitation costs and actual costs; *see also care system model, and direct contracting*

provider HMO—often used to include any HMO that is either the result of a provider decision to become an HMO (with normal licensure application and approval), a PSN, or a retail HMO (but does not include a private label HMO, which involves a leased license from an existing HMO); *see also HMO, private label HMO, PSN, and retail HMO*

provider inpatient cost control—the admitting physician or inpatient physician is able to impact the utilization of resources to some degree, relating to the site of admission, types and quantity of supplies, tests and services for laboratory or X-ray, added consultations with specialists, medications prescribed, and the timing of discharge or transfer to a transitional bed or any other type of lower cost alternative; the management of care utilization alternatives focuses education on these choices, with the goal of reducing cost while maintaining a quality outcome; *see also physician unit cost hospital pool, and standing orders*

provider–insurer alliance or partnership—*see ODS, second definition*

provider network—not necessarily a PSN (since PSN entities represent only a proposed formation that could enter into risk relationships in lieu of formally licensed HMOs), and may be a group of providers supporting a particular payer, or as a separate, non-HMO network that is capable of providing support; a provider network is either the reference to the number of providers, the specialty mix, and the geographic distribution, which is hopefully attractive for award of federal or commercial payer business; *see also PSN*

provider network exclusion safeguards—*see exclusion safeguards*

provider profiling—the collection of provider utilization information including cost per admission, pharmaceutical and specialist utilization, and other parameters that would give an

indication of medical practice habits; profiling may be conducted by entities as large as an HMO or as small as a pod-level group of providers at risk, to ensure that a provider under consideration of being added to the network or pod shows practice behavior conducive to managed care, and the ability to control downstream costs that detract from earnings; *see also downstream costs, and profiling*

provider RFP—provider Request for Proposal; a strategy for providers to turn the table on payers, perhaps using their strength in the market to solicit payer responses to a Request for Proposal, which contains payer estimates of the volume of patients, medical services requested, and the pricing offered by the payer; some providers use this technique to gain semi-exclusive arrangements with a few strong payer partners who offer higher payment; *see also semi-exclusive contract*

provider service network—another way of defining a provider-sponsored network; *see PSO*

provider service quality—*see physician service quality; see also physician patient retention program*

provider-sponsored network—*see PSN*

prudent layperson—as state and federal governments have introduced legislation to narrow the definition of "emergency services," many bills have expressed them as services that any prudent layperson would judge as a true emergency; if they are deemed to be emergency services, then they are reimbursed, regardless of whether a true emergency actually existed; some fear that a wider interpretation allows health costs to increase; *see also emergency, and emergency services*

PSN—provider-sponsored network; *see PSO*

PSO—provider-sponsored organization; formal affiliation of providers, organized to provide a substantial portion of health care services; a term used in the Balanced Budget Act of 1997 for the Medicare+Choice program; PSOs contract with Medicare as public or private entities, HMOs, PPOs, fee-for-service, and Medical Savings Account plans; *see also direct contracting, HMO, ODS, private label HMO, provider HMO, and retail HMO*

PSRO—Professional Standards Review Organization; under Medicare and Medicaid programs, these organizations function as the PRO to ensure medical necessity and professional standards of care; *see also PRO*

PTMPY—per thousand members per year; normally used by hospitals to calculate the utilization of services

public entity—used within the context of employee health benefit plans for qualified HMOs to include the 50 states, Puerto Rico, Guam, the Virgin Islands, and Northern Mariana Islands and American Samoa and their political subdivisions, the District of Columbia, and any agency of the above; *see also political subdivision*

public hospital—hospital operated by state, county, or local government and often viewed as the facility of last resort for charity care patients; likely to receive and treat patients transferred by patient dumping from other hospitals in the area; often the public hospital's tax exempt status due to its community support becomes a target by other for-profit hospitals or hospital chains, which point out the degree of their contributions to the community, while lobbying for the tax exempt status of competitors to be removed

purchasing alliance—a group of health care purchasers that may be private, public, or combinations of both (contrasted with health insurance purchasing cooperatives that tend to support a governmental entity), brought together with a purpose of a strengthened negotiating position as one entity in dealing with one or more health plans; one state purchasing alliance has formed in California for a group of employers, another in Kentucky for employers, public groups, and individuals, with other structures in Iowa and Florida—other states are also considering formations; purchasing agents within the alliance attempt to find the best price and quality within a geographical area; this approach may be the solution to give small busi-

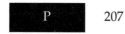

nesses the group contract access and market clout needed; *see also HIPC, and hospital alliance*

purchasing coalition—*see purchasing alliance*

purchasing cooperative—*see purchasing alliance*

pure indemnity—*see indemnity; see also managed indemnity*

Q

QARI—Quality Assurance Reform Initiative; a collaborative effort by HCFA, states, the managed care industry, and consumer advocates to design practical approaches to monitoring and improving the quality of Medicaid managed care services; in 1995 QARI published Health Care Quality Improvement Studies in Managed Care, together with NCQA; *see also HCFA, and NCQA*

QI—quality improvement; a management engineering theory that lends itself well to the medical industry for obtaining continuous and incremental improvements, identifies problems in health care delivery, tests solutions to those problems, and tracks implemented solutions; QI seeks to identify the optimal process to accomplish a task and then eliminate process deviation that brings either waste or delay; QI is also called linear improvement, as opposed to the "clean sheet of paper" approach to the more nonlinear theory of reengineering, which allows the team to design a preferred process as if no process were already in place; also called continuous quality improvement (CQI), total quality management (TQM), quality management (QM), or total quality improvement (TQI); *see also patient care reengineering*

QMB—qualified Medicare beneficiary; the qualification for Medicare is determined by the Social Security Administration to see who is entitled to receive Medicare benefits, based on factors such as age 65 or older, people of any age with permanent kidney failure, and certain disabled people under 65; a beneficiary may be qualified for hospital insurance under Part A, or optionally qualified for medical insurance under Part B; *see also Medicare*

qualified HMO—an HMO found by HCFA to be qualified within the meaning of section 1310 of the PHS Act and subpart D as either an operational, preoperational, or transitional qualified HMO; *see also federal qualification, operational qualified HMO, preoperational qualified HMO, or transitionally qualified HMO*

qualified Medicare beneficiary—*see QMB*

quality adjusted life-year—measurement unit to define health outcomes that result from medical or surgical care, expressed in terms of the number of years of life in a less-desirable health condition as compared to years of full health; if the estimated quality of life for a bedridden patient is 50% with a life expectancy of 10 years, the measurement would be 5 quality adjusted life-years; to the extent that the U.S. system of medicine becomes more focused on termination of life when the quality of life or chances of long-term survival is low, more attention will be given to this measurement

quality assurance—program activities that are conducted from the perspective of individual hospitals or insurers, as reviewed by internal leadership or external entities such as NCQA, to ensure that medical care and service meet clinical standards of quality; recurring agenda items for formal meetings as well as interim studies include elements of peer review and audits of care, medical protocols, credentialing, and assessment of patient satisfaction; *see also medical protocols, NCQA, QI, and UM*

Quality Assurance Reform Initiative—*see QARI*

quality improvement—*see QI*

quasi-SNF—a level of skilled nursing facility (commonly pronounced "SNIFF") that is between a SNF and acute care hospitalization; a setting for care that is more cost-effective than an extended hospital stay, yet requires more care and staffing than a SNF; quasi-SNF nurse staffing can be augmented with aides and LPNs, and does not require 24-hour physician coverage; *see also SNF, and transitional bed*

quota law for primary care—*see PCP quota law*

R&C—reasonable and customary; the amount of money usually billed for health care services within a given region; sometimes all fees in the 80th or 90th percentile are averaged to determine R&C, and other times R&C is synonymous with fees schedule rate ceilings, when the rates are relatively high; *see also prevailing charge*

range of services—used to define the prepaid arrangements to provide basic health services, as an operationally qualified HMO; *see basic health services*

RAPS—Resource Analysis & Planning System; an interactive, on-line computer analysis tool, developed and maintained by the Defense Medical Information System program, and used to forecast both military and dependent population data, and MTF inpatient and outpatient workload data up to five years into the future; RAPS also estimates the subset of actual users for MTF, to support planning, policy, and operational decisions for the Department of Defense

rate—*see premium*

rate bands—*see adjusted community rating, and community rating by class*

rate setting—*see all-payer rate setting*

rating process—within the health plan or HMO, an evaluation takes place to determine what premium should be charged for a particular group or individual; the analysis considers the type of risk inherent and applies known values for the age and sex mix factors, geographic location, type of industry in which the employees are involved, base capitation factor, the actual design of the plan including copays and deductibles (which gives the experienced analyst good assumptions regarding how likely patients are to use the plan), average family size, demographics, and costs that will be charged against the plan

RBE—risk-bearing entity; a legal entity that is structured to assume some portion of risk associated with managed care, through its funding and insurance protection, such as an LLC, or a managed care organization

RBRVS—resource-based relative value scale; a system used initially by Medicare for physician reimbursement, but with spin-off influence on other sectors, to more properly assess the skill and resource relationships to specific CPT codes; RBRVS is adjusted for regional deviations, related charges, and overhead; the resulting scale was developed to compensate for Medicare's tendency to overpay for procedural services such as surgery and diagnostic tests, while underpaying for cognitive primary care services involving examination and discussion/education with patients; three conversion factors are currently used for surgical, primary care, and all other services; a congressional proposal tried to create a single conversion factor in 1996, but RBRVS would still be used for FFS Medicare; *see also MVPS, and SGR*

readmission review—review of patients readmitted to a hospital within seven days with problems related to the first admission, to determine whether the first discharge was premature and/or the second admission is medically necessary

real value—used in health economics to measure the value after adjustment for inflation over time, so that the result is a constant dollar or measurement

reasonable and customary charge—*see R&C*

reasonable charges (Medicare definition)—within the context of Medicare Part B, this is the basis of payment for medical services and certain other health services; the reasonable charge is the lowest of either the actual charge billed by the physician or supplier, the charge the physician or supplier customarily bills

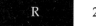
patients for the same service, or the prevailing charge most physicians or suppliers in that locality bill for the same service

recipient—associated with a person who meets the requirements to be eligible for Medicaid

recurring claim provision—a provision in some health insurance policies that specifies a length of time during which the recurrence of a condition is considered to be a continuation of a previous period of disability or hospital confinement

redirecting patients—*see channeling, and exclusivity*

reduction of payments—if an HMO or CMP requests a reduction in its monthly payments (because it has an ACR less than the average of the per capita rates of payment and it has requested a reduction in monthly payment instead of offering its enrollees added benefits), HCFA will reduce payments accordingly; reductions may also be made for election of hospital or SNF payment options

reengineering—*see patient care reengineering*

referral—the request for additional care, usually of a specialty nature as requested by a primary care physician or another specialist needing additional medical information on behalf of the patient; referrals within the context of managed care are more restricted in the sense that a PCP who accepts financial risk for downstream medical care is more sensitive to the balance between medical necessity and cost; good information systems are needed to track referral costs that aid physicians in learning more about this factor; *see also downstream costs*

referral provider—any provider receiving a referral as defined above, such as a specialist who is asked to provide more insight regarding the medical problems of a patient who is being referred from a family physician, gatekeeper, or any PCP of a plan

referral services—those eligible hospital services that, due to the specialized nature of the service or facility required, are not available and cannot be provided by a participating provider; these services must be specifically authorized by the plan before the services are rendered

refinement—used to describe the adjustment of incorrect Medicare relative value scale; *see also RVS*

regional IDN—an integrated delivery network for an entire region; *see IDN*

regional integrated systems of care—the focus of existing health provider systems, developing further toward becoming regional systems of care, has been energized by language within the draft American Health Security Act, and also through the award of CHAMPUS regional contracts, and the creation of the Department of Veteran Affairs VISNs

rehabilitation (rehab)—process and goal of restoring disabled members to maximum physical, mental, and vocational independence and productivity; achieved by identifying and developing residual capabilities, job modification, or retraining; rehab provision language is present in some long-term disability policies that allow for benefits or other financial assistance to continue during the rehab period

rehabilitation facility—an institution licensed as a rehabilitation facility by the laws of the state where it is located, and which: is operated within the scope of its license, provides 24-hour nursing care furnished or supervised by RNs, maintains daily clinical records on each patient, has the services of a physician available at all time under an established agreement, uses appropriate methods to dispense and administer drugs and medicines, has transfer arrangements with at least one hospital, has a utilization review plan in effect, and has treatment policies developed with the advice of (and reviewed by) a group of professionals who are specialists in the care and treatment provided by the institution

reimbursable costs—allowable costs are determined according to a formula negotiated by the hospital and HMO; the HMO

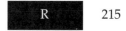

then reimburses the hospital retrospectively, based on the costs incurred according to the agreed-on formula

reinstatement—resumption of coverage under a policy that had lapsed

reinsurance—insurance to guard against the partial or complete loss of money from medical claims, which may be procured by policyholders who are either insurance companies themselves, or providers, or employers; typical coverage is purchased for either individual stop loss, aggregate stop loss, out-of-area care, and insolvency protection; a larger health plan typically reduces reinsurance coverage as it grows; *see also risk control insurance, and stop loss insurance*

relative value method—any type of payment methodology that assigns a unit value to a procedure, multiplied by some conversion factor, which establishes interrelationships among procedures; not currently a method for payment between any known purchaser and commercial HMO (versus the fee for service, discounted FFS, and multiple capitation methods), but used internally by some HMOs to pay physicians; Medicare uses one example called RBRVS; *see also DFFS, FFS, and RBRVS*

relative value scale—*see RVS*

relative weighted product—a measure used in health care cost accounting and data analysis that works to link the amount of personnel time, medical resources, and cost involved to care for a DRG; the higher the RWP, the more hospital resources are required to care for that illness or injury

renewal—the decision or act of keeping a health care policy after the expiration of its initial period of coverage, by continuing to pay premium amounts that have been determined by the insurers as the rates for the upcoming term

replacement insurance—insurance that replaces the coverage under a particular health policy with coverage under another policy

reserve—*see PCR*

reserves—fiscal method of providing a fund for incurred but not reported health services or other financial liabilities; also refers to deposits and/or other financial requirements that must be met by an entity as defined by various state or federal regulatory authorities

residual disability benefits—benefits within an insurance policy that provide funds in proportion to the reduction of earnings as a result of disability, versus the inability to work full-time

Resource Analysis & Planning System—*see RAPS*

resource-based relative value scale—*see RBRVS*

Resource Sharing—the CHAMPUS TRICARE feature within the new regional series of DoD managed care support contracts that encourages dialogue between a DoD military treatment facility and the HMO to determine any mutual benefit of sharing staff, equipment, maintenance services, or supplies; internal resource sharing supplements MTF services, while external resource sharing allows care at a network facility; *see also CHAMPUS, and TRICARE*

respite care—entitlement for short-term child care to allow a parent to get relief, or prevent child abuse; or care in the absence of a regular caregiver that involves a short hospice stay to give temporary relief to a person who regularly assists with home care

respondent superior—the legal doctrine of vicarious liability, which may be applied in the case of a suit against a health care provider by a patient, making the employer responsible for the employee's negligent acts, because the employer has the right to control this behavior

retail HMO—the entity created after a decision by a provider to gain an HMO license (through lease from an existing HMO, or purchase in accordance with state insurance commission rules)

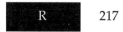

and enter the direct retail relationships and responsibilities to the consumer or employer/purchaser (as opposed to providing health care on a wholesale basis to the consumer or employer/purchaser through another HMO); essentially an HMO with a license; *see also HMO, and provider HMO*

retail hospital marketing—a strategy of marketing directly to consumers, from the perspective of a hospital or provider network, versus wholesale marketing to insurers; may be performed in order to inform employers or patients of the hospital's value and essential role in their care, or to persuade them that they do not need to use an HMO, or even to protest that an HMO is planning to exclude them from a network; *see also exclusivity, PSN, and wholesale hospital marketing*

retention—another way of describing the administrative fee that normally serves as the profit that keeps the plan "in the black," or retained earnings; retention funds may be either reinvested in the company, applied toward the cost of medical claims and miscellaneous expenses, or in the case of for-profit companies, they are passed to shareholders; *see also MLR*

retention of members—*see patient retention*

retirement center—*see retirement residence*

retirement residence—organized program or community living environment that provides social services and activities to retired persons who generally require almost no assistance or ongoing health care; also called independent or congregate living; designed specifically for independent senior adults; services usually include (but in some cases optional) meals, housekeeping, and laundry; social activities are usually entertaining and educational and help to foster a great sense of community among the residents; less health service than an assisted living center

retro add—retroactive additions to a capitation list; for example when a member became effectively added for insurance coverage on January 1st, but does not appear on the capitation list until April 1st at which point the error is noticed, the member months for this member will require a retro add of three months and a correction of payment

retro delete—retroactive deletions to a capitation list, for example when a member terminates health plan coverage on January 1st, but continues to appear on the capitation list until April 1st at which point the error is noticed, the plan must perform a retro delete of three member months and a correction of payment

retrospective review—a method of determining medical necessity, quality of care, and/or appropriate billing practice for services that have already been rendered; the trend is moving away from retrospective review and toward concurrent review of admissions, in order to preclude unnecessary treatment and cost; *see also concurrent review, and prospective review*

revenue—premium proceeds paid from individual enrollees, groups, or employers to a health plan in return for health care of covered members and all specified support or information infrastructure services; *see also premium*

revenue share—the portion of revenue devoted to one type of health product, or type of expense, which is expressed as a percent of overall revenue

reverse RFP—reverse Request for Proposal; sometimes used to describe a provider-initiated RFP; *see provider RFP*

RF network—radio frequency network; *see wireless technology*

rightsizing—using market forces of supply and demand to determine pricing or capacity; may apply to the "right" number of beds within a facility, the right number of outpatient clinics within a metropolitan area, or the right price to pay for specialty capitation, based on market rates

risk—any likelihood of loss foreseen by a provider, IDN, or insurer in providing health care services; also refers to the

generic arrangements within managed care that involve a departure from FFS medicine toward prepayment, which focuses on the care of a given population by a primary care provider or hospital system taking full economic responsibility for that population's care needs; *see also covered lives, and PCR*

risk adjuster—a means of compensating for health spending costs of a particular patient population that are projected to be higher or lower than the average health demographics, by adjusting the payment to an insurer based on the risk for these enrollees; *see also risk adjustment*

risk adjuster model—pilot projects have been developed as alternative methods of payment arrangement, which use either Ambulatory Care Groups as an outpatient classification scheme for HCFA on Medicare risk (as in Johns Hopkins and Lewin/VHI, Inc.), or the DCG approach (by Boston University and the Center for Health Economics Research); risk adjuster models are encouraged for Medicare Choices

risk adjustment—may refer to a generic system to adjust for, or distribute the risk of Medicare enrollees, such as AAPCC; or risk adjustment administrative policies that do not allow HMOs to refuse enrollment to an individual because of a medical condition, review by HCFA of marketing and recruitment by an HMO, mandate for an annual 30-day open enrollment period, or the allowance for beneficiaries to disenroll at any time after written notice; may include reinsurance strategies; more comprehensive risk adjustment models are being sought by some to include some measure of health status; *see also AAPCC, adverse selection, favorable selection, open enrollment period, reinsurance, and risk adjuster model*

risk analysis—the methodology for evaluation of the expected medical care costs for a prospective group, which also involves the best application of all available products (with the employer-customer in mind), to include benefit levels and prices that best meet the needs of the group under evaluation

risk-bearing entity—*see RBE*

risk-bearing PPO—HCFA's description of one possible construction for the Medicare Choices demonstration project that
entails blended risk payments, use of a network of providers
and hospitals who have agreed to accept negotiated prices for
both Part A and Part B Medicare services, and to use a designated UM program; *see also Medicare Choices demonstration
project, and PPO*

risk contract—a generic description of a contract involving medical claims risk on a prepayment basis between two entities,
such as a provider and an HMO, HCFA and a federally qualified HMO, or an integrated delivery network and an individual PCP or medical group; the risk contract will specify the
medical services to be included, together with the associated
reimbursement structure, the amount of withhold or physician
contingency reserve to be set aside for potential claims above
estimates, or incremental risk corridors; if claims run above
projections, it is the responsibility of the party that bears risk
under the contract to pay those excess costs, whereas any savings is similarly given to the party bearing risk; Medicare risk
contracts are presently used by 9% of eligibles versus FFS
Medicare; *see also Medicare Choices demonstration project, PCR,
reinsurance, risk, and risk corridor*

risk control insurance—*see reinsurance*

risk corridor—a mechanism that allows contract performance
within ranges of financial performance, or corridors, in order
to apply risk as specifically stated; such as the case where providers work within the corridor of actual claims per member
per month, and are released if claims expenses fall above the
corridor, or may be rewarded below the corridor (so for a 10%
corridor on a PCP set at $23 PMPM, the physician will be sub-
ject to rewards for amounts under $21.70); risk corridors have
many formats to incentivize performance accordingly

risk factor—in this case, the health factors related to disease,
which may be either established factors (i.e., heredity, sex, race,
and age) or factors that are influenced by behavior (smoking,
inactivity, or response to stress); with the growth of managed

care, health plans and systems are learning the outpatient and inpatient costs of various diseases, and the average total monthly claims costs per covered life for hypertension, atherosclerosis, etc.; the goal of current studies or programs is to promote behavior that reduces the cost of care for populations; *see health promotion*

risk HMOs/CMPs—language used by HCFA to describe a federally qualified HMO or competitive medical plan that assumes all the financial risk of caring for Medicare beneficiaries through their provider networks; Medicare pays risk HMOs or CMPs a per capita premium for an agreed-upon package of benefits (see cost HMOs for an alternative comparison of adjustments at the end of the year for variations from the budget); added benefits of prescription drugs and eyeglasses may be added; members must receive all of their care through the HMO or CMP network, except for emergency and out-of-area urgent care; these are appealing plans to Medicare beneficiaries who seek comprehensive, quality care for the least out-of-pocket expense and minimal paperwork

risk management—a health care function or discipline that executes one or more strategies to limit the organization to the financial risk associated with delivering care; may include the strategy of reviewing the actuarial risk of a given enrollment population toward catastrophic care, purchasing insurance or self-insuring to protect against risk, associated medico-legal factors to protect against undue risk, or organizational programs to preclude the occurrence of health events that typically lead to legal claims; *see also risk adjustment*

risk pool—*see pool*

risk selection—may result in either favorable selection or adverse selection when insurers (or enrollees) take intentional or unintentional action to enroll members (or sign up for coverage) resulting in an unequal distribution of risk as compared to the population as a whole; also called biased selection; *see also adverse selection, and favorable selection*

risk sharing—a generic term used to define any mechanism that gives financial incentive to managed care providers for rendering cost-effective, high-quality care; *see also pool*

routine inpatient services—hospital room and board and related professional services for which, generally, there is no separate charge, because specialty care is not needed beyond this basic provision

routine physicals—a typical service included within a risk HMO contract; *see additional benefits to Medicare risk*

rule-based protocol—a type of health care delivery protocol, not including the area of medical protocols, which establishes universal rules to: apply case management to all potentially large cases, perform tests prior to standard admissions, mandatory use of PCP for referrals, and second opinions prior to routine surgery; *see also medical protocols*

rural area—any area not listed as a place having a population of 2,500 or more in the "Number of Inhabitants" Document PC(1)A of Table VI "Population of Places" and not listed as an urbanized area in Table XI "Population of Urbanized Areas" of the most recent update of the Bureau of Census, U.S. Department of Commerce

RVS—relative value scale; the Medicare scale that assigns weights to each medical service, in terms of the relative amount to be paid for that service; the three components of the RVS are the value of the physician's work (or Work Relative Value), the expense to the physician's practice, and the relative amount of physician malpractice expense for that service; *see also RBRVS, and WRV*

RVU—relative value unit; the building block of RBRVS; for each service, there are three RVUs to cover work, practice expenses, and the cost of professional liability insurance

RWP—*see relative weighted product*

safety net providers—another name for Community Health Centers; *see CHC*

salaried physician—a physician who is compensated solely from a monthly or annual salary, as in a staff model HMO, federal, or military physician employment; no reimbursement is given for other factors, such as utilization efficiency, production, percentage of medical group profits, or physician contingency reserve bonus; *see also PCR, physician production formula, and staff model HMO*

same day surgery—*see ASC*

sanction—occurs when a health plan finds it necessary to reprimand a participating provider, for reasons outlined according to standards of conduct or acceptable behavior within the plan

saturation—a market-related term used to describe an HMO's achievement of maximum enrollment likely within a given market area or service area

scored savings—a projection or scoring by the Congressional Budget Office for a particular piece of proposed health legislation

SCR—standard class rate; a revenue requirements-oriented projection tool for PMPM calculation within a group demographic setting, which is used to determine monthly insurance premium rates that will be charged for a particular group; *see also ASR*

screening—a practice used by HMOs to limit access to care for those requests that are not medically necessary; *see also gatekeeper model*

screening measures—rate-based indicators of the effectiveness of the plan's efforts to screen a targeted population for early detection of a specific disease

secondary care—the specialty medical care or services provided by a referral provider; *see also gatekeeper model, PCP, and referral provider*

secondary coverage—refers to the plan or policy that must pay for any medical care or services that the primary payer is not required to reimburse; any insurance such as privately purchased Medigap, Medicaid, or employer coverage that supplements Medicare; Medicare is the secondary payer when the beneficiary has other primary insurance, or when reimbursement will be obtained from third-party liability; *see also COB, MG policy, and primary coverage*

secondary insurance—*see secondary coverage*

secondary payer—*see secondary coverage*

SELECT—*see Medicare SELECT*

selective contracting—a contentious strategy or mechanism between providers and insurers that allows managed care organizations to select only the best physicians, in terms of practice utilization, training, etc., versus using any willing provider (in federal or commercial managed care); seen as a cost control measure by the insurer, a "right to practice" issue by physicians, and a consumer choice issue by patient organizations; generally supported by the FTC; *see also AWP, exclusivity, and PPA*

self-care—an approach or philosophy that views the patient as the primary care provider, as well as the consumer of health care; calls for a variety of health education strategies that enable the patient to become competent with self-diagnosis and treatment for an estimated range of 70-90% of all symptoms, yielding reduced visits for ambulatory care or minor illness

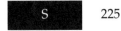

self-funded health plan—*see self-insurance*

self-funding—*see self-insurance*

self-insurance—a risk strategy that allows the potential profit that an HMO or carrier traditionally receives from funding insurance risk to be experienced instead by an employer (or other legal entity, which may be a hospital-based delivery network) rather than an HMO; contrasted from reinsurance, in that an external insurance protection is not used as a general format, but certain protection may be sought for segments such as catastrophic; essentially, the health benefits are funded from internal resources without purchasing insurance; self-insurance entities may obtain outside administrative assistance to manage requirements; *see also reinsurance, and stop loss*

self-insured health plan—*see self-insurance*

self-referral restriction—state-level legislation has augmented the federal restrictions covered within the Stark I and Stark II laws guarding against provider self-referral, with over 30 states setting limits that run the spectrum from narrow to truly broad restrictions; *see also Stark I, and Stark II*

semi-exclusive contract—a contractual arrangement by a payer to allow only two (or a limited number of) providers in the network, or for the provider to contract with a specified limit of payers, in return for price concessions or other favorable terms that warrant the limitation; often used when a totally exclusive arrangement is not reasonable, or is potentially hazardous to either party, considering the geographical coverage requirements or local market competition; some semi-exclusive contracts have a release clause, assuming certain conditions do not materialize, such as a minimum level of enrollment or performance; *see also exclusivity, and provider RFP*

senior advisor—*see Medicare senior representative*

senior care—any segment or market that is targeted to emphasize health care services for the growing number of senior citizens, such as assisted living centers, LTC, nursing homes, retirement housing, or specific managed care products for the 65 and older population; *see also Medicare risk*

senior care ambassador—*see Medicare senior representative*

senior care outreach—*see geriatric outreach*

service area—the specific region in which health care services are conducted and outlined for approval by a state insurance regulator as of the effective date of the agreement; within an IDN context, the service area is the local area that the network considers not only to be its immediate market area but also the approximate borderline that may constitute agreement with nearby provider systems for noncompetition according to an agreement, or in the absence of an agreement may be openly competed between one IDN and another, through the placement of PCPs or other tactics; if during the course of an agreement, the service area expands to a new geographical area, then the new area is deemed to comprise the service area; *see also significant expansion*

service benefit contract—a contract that provides the covered services themselves rather than providing reimbursement for some or all of the expenses the subscriber incurs in obtaining covered services

service plan—a health insurance plan involving direct contracts with providers but not necessarily managed care, such as Blue Cross and Blue Shield contracts involving direct billing to the plan by providers and direct payment by the plan to providers; in exchange for the efficiencies that result from direct relationships between provider and plan, the providers agree to accept certain rates and payment in full, with no balance billing to the patient; may address quality of care and utilization

service quality measures—indicators of whether enrollees believe that their health plan or provider is responsive, accessible, pleasant, "user friendly," punctual, and respectful of their needs; with the relative difficulty of differentiating the quality

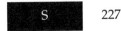
of care between plans or providers, service quality is an important factor that customers can assess and then make enrollment or disenrollment decisions based on their judgment; *see also physician service quality*

service reimbursement system—a term used to define the Medicare tradition of reimbursing for a stated level of services; versus a premium support system, or a futuristic Medicare system that shifts emphasis to having the government pay a certain portion of an insurance policy premium for a beneficiary; *see also premium support system*

set aside—under proposed MediGrant procedures (which may change before this printing), states would be required to establish set aside funds to cover four groups: elderly, disabled, low-income families, and Medicare/MediGrant dual eligibles; set asides have been drafted to require 85% of the average FY92 to FY94 expenditure for each group; federal funds for each state were capped beginning in FY96, with a certain percent of maximum growth rate to be specified for later payment years; *see also Medicaid, and MediGrant*

seventy-five twenty-five test or 75-25 rule—the 75-25 test is a federal regulation that requires an HMO servicing Medicaid patients to have a current enrollment of at least 25% of commercial patients; changes may be likely in this area as active state-level Medicaid projects cause policy to be reevaluated

SGR—sustainable growth rate; a system proposed within the congressional reconciliation package on Medicare reform as a replacement for the current MVPS, which would essentially tie the level of government payment to a calculation that reflects what the market will sustain; the SGR would use an MVPS-type conversion factor based on enrollment volume, plus changes in the Medicare Economic Index (MEI), and changes in gross domestic product plus 2%, with updates limited to a fail-safe mechanism of no more than 103% and no less than 93% of MEI; *see also MEI, MVPS, PPRC, and RBRVS*

shadow pricing—the practice of setting premium rates at a level equal or just below the competition's rates whether or not those rates can be justified—generally considered to be unethical and illegal

share of cost—under Medicaid, patients must pay their share of cost each month before they can be eligible for Medicaid coverage; also called liability or spend down

shared risk—an arrangement where any two entities, such as a health plan and a provider, agree to share in the risk to some contracted percentage of hospital costs that may come in over budget, but also allows the sharing of profits for care provided under budget; *see also pool, and risk sharing*

Sherman Act—(15 U.S.C., 1&2) establishes safeguards against health entities forming monopolies, restraint of trade, price fixing, or commerce conspiracy; strategies that contain an anticompetitive outcome or market power to control prices by acquisition are problematic, which leaves the course of being better and smarter as competitors as the only safe method for growth; *see also antitrust laws, and Clayton Act*

short-stay hospital—a category of general and special hospitals that average less than 30 days ALOS for patients

short-term disability income insurance—a provision to pay benefits to a covered disabled person as long as he or she remains disabled, up to a specified period of time not exceeding two years

significant business transaction—any business transaction or series of transactions during any one fiscal year of the HMO, the total value of which exceeds the lesser of $25,000 or 5% of the total operating expenses of the HMO; significant business transactions must be reported to HCFA annually, within 120 days after the end of the fiscal year (unless extended by HCFA) for any: sale, exchange, or lease of property; loan of money or extension of credit; or goods, services, or facilities furnished for a monetary consideration

significant expansion—a planned substantial increase in the enrollment of the HMO that requires an increase in the number

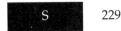

of health professionals serving enrollees of the HMO, or an expansion of the physician capacity of the HMO's total health facilities; a planned expansion of the service area beyond the current service area that would be made possible by adding health service delivery facilities and health professionals to serve enrollees at a new site or sites in areas previously without service sites; *see also expansion of services, and service area*

similar area—an area similar to the HMO's or CMP's geographic area but free from special characteristics that would distort the determination of the AAPCC

single-carrier replacement—occurs when a purchaser drops existing carriers currently in place and covers all eligible members through one carrier

single-payer health system—a centralized delivery system such as Canada's, in which the government pays the bills for health care; any physician or hospital may be used for care; the government would set prices and impose regulations, but doctors, hospitals, and other providers would remain in the private sector

site-of-service differential—a payment schedule that provides different levels of reimbursement, depending upon the site of service; designed to reward the lowest cost site setting that is appropriate for a particular type of patient care of service, yet provide patient choice

site visit—the second step of HCFA's procedures to federally qualify an HMO or CMP, in which the HCFA team visits the candidate for two days to verify information provided in the application, to explore issues in depth, conduct interviews, and specifically review finances, marketing, health services delivery, and legal systems; at a closing session the team identifies any added information needed to finalize review and issues a 14-day suspense for the return of this added information to HCFA

skilled care—the level of care that requires the services of a registered nurse on a regular basis for treatments and procedures;

skilled care also includes services provided by specially trained professionals, such as physical and respiratory therapists; *see also SNF*

skilled nursing facility—*see SNF*

skimming—efforts by an insurer to gain favorable selection; state and federal governments are attempting to level the playing field against skimming through guaranteed issue, guaranteed renewal, and portability; *see also favorable selection, guaranteed issue, guaranteed renewal, and portability*

sliding price scale—a range of prices is available under a sliding scale, with better pricing (using the example of hospital discounts) in exchange for a preferred status or increased volume (such as an HMO that agrees to limit the number of hospitals in its network)

small group pooling—used by many carriers to combine small businesses into a pool to spread risk; some states have pioneered formal opportunities for statewide pools to support small businesses that could not otherwise provide group coverage for their employees

small subscriber group aggregate—*see small group pooling*

smart card—a wallet-sized card that contains medical history for use by the Columbia/HCA Healthcare Corporation; *see also EMR*

SMI—supplemental medical insurance; also known as Medicare Part B; a voluntary insurance program for aged and disabled persons who elect to enroll; provides insurance benefits for physician and other medical services under Title 18 of the Social Security Act; nearly 95% of eligible people are enrolled through the payment of a monthly premium and a matching amount from the federal government; after the annual deductible has been met, SMI pays for 80% of the reasonable charge for most covered services—this coverage includes physician services, home health care, medical and other health services,

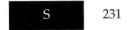

outpatient hospital services, laboratory, pathology, and radiology; *see also Medicare Part B*

SNF—skilled nursing facility (commonly pronounced "SNIF"); a setting for care that was designed to be more cost-effective than an extended hospital stay; a facility, either freestanding or part of a hospital, that accepts patients in need of rehab or needing 24-hour skilled nursing; SNFs also have access to a full range of therapy for speech, physical, and occupational applications; SNFs and sub-acute care facilities are an important aspect for cost constraint, compared to traditional hospitalization; *see also observation unit, quasi-SNF, sub-acute care, and transitional bed*

SOAP—the method of documenting medical records or progress notes with S for subjective complaints, O for objective findings, A for assessment of status, and P for the diagnostic or therapeutic plan; used as a standard for medical records documentation both in and out of managed care settings

social HMO—federally funded Medicare demonstration project for the elderly; provides comprehensive health and long-term care benefits to Medicare beneficiaries; unlike other Medicare-enrolling HMOs, care in a social HMO is reimbursed at 100%

socialized medicine—differentiated from national health insurance in that this system is always regulated and controlled by the government, with government responsibility for providing health and hospital care of the entire population, at no direct cost or at a nominal fee to the individual, by means of subsidies obtained through taxes

SPD—summary plan description; the list of covered benefits for an employee, which must be provided in writing to all members within a self-funded health insurance plan

specialist channeling—the practice by a plan, provider, medical group, or pod-level risk entity, to direct referrals to a single specialist, or to a small number of cost-effective specialists and away from others that do not practice quality care with appropriate utilization in the judgment of the channeler; patient volume increases for the specialists receiving channeling, and downstream costs are hopefully reduced; effective channeling to providers must be done as a result of good cost information for individual specialists within specialty areas; *see also physician channeling, and specialist deselection*

specialist deselection—the elimination of certain specialists from a network or plan, based on their high cost or unwillingness to work with managed care models; occurs in the more advanced markets, and allows a greater number of patients for each remaining specialist who is not eliminated; deselection may cause negative comments from patients or the community, while also limiting network coverage; *see also channeling*

specialist referral authorization—all referrals of system or plan enrollees to participating specialists, including those made by phone, must be authorized in writing by the enrollee's PCP

specialty capitation—a system of payment that provides a capitated payment for specialty care, according to one of many reimbursement methods; the PMPM amount is determined through negotiation, but is based on the actuarial determination of specialty care utilization costs for a comparable sample of patients; a portion of the capitation payment may be a withhold; *see also chronic care capitation, contact capitation, PCR, and specialty department capitation*

specialty capitation–individual—*see individual specialtist capitation*

specialty contact capitation—*see contact capitation*

specialty coverage—most contracts between insurers and employers outline minimum provider network requirements for specialties as either: access on a ratio of specialists per 1,000 patient population enrolled, one-way driving distance for the patient, or other minimum specialties and subspecialties as listed

specialty department capitation—involves capitating a specialty at the department level, with a payment to be divided among the number of physicians in the department; considered sub-optimal because it still allows churning, with more billing for more services rendered, which may include more inpatient uti-lization; individual specialists avoid lower incomes by increas-ing utilization to gain a larger share; some negative effects are limited in small groups with extensive communication and col-legiality; *see also contact capitation, and individual specialist capita-tion*

specialty managed care—*see niche service*

specialty networks—another name for horizontally integrated networks; *see also horizontal integration*

specified disease insurance—insurance providing an unallo-cated benefit, subject to a maximum amount, for expenses incurred in connection with the treatment of specified diseases, such as cancer, poliomyelitis, encephalitis, and spinal meningi-tis; these policies are designed to supplement major medical policies

SPIN—standard prescriber identification number; a unique iden-tifier that is currently under development for future use to sup-port prescribing providers, in an effort be headed by the National Council of Prescription Drug Programs and other professional organizations

sponsor—the primary employee or enrolled member for whom coverage is provided (aside from any specific consideration for dependent insurance); within CHAMPUS terminology, the sponsor is the military service member, either active duty, retired, or deceased, whose relationship makes the patient eli-gible for care

SSA—the Social Security Administration, which administers Social Security Disability Insurance (SSDI) and Supplemental Security Income (SSI) for disabled or self-employed persons

SSI—Supplemental Security Income; a program of income support for low-income, aged, blind, and disabled persons established in Title 16 of the Social Security Act

staff model enrollment equity—an analytical system that aids staff model HMOs to determine the number of patients that can be managed by a PCP; serves as an objective mechanism to ensure an equitable distribution, in salary-based systems that have no added incentives for increased production performance; may include factors and weights for age/sex distribution, maternity care, inpatient rounding workload, and psychiatric care

staff model HMO—an HMO model that enters into a relationship with its physicians as employees, in order to provide health care to its members; premiums are paid to the HMO, which in turn pays providers as staff members; increasingly, the staff models are exploring new incentive pay structures, versus a flat salary that may not properly incentivize desired behaviors; normally PCPs within this model are not allowed to have a large portion of FFS patients; considered by some as the most efficient managed care model; *see also group model HMO*

staff of the HMO—health professionals who are employees of the HMO and who: provide services to HMO enrollees at an HMO facility subject to the staff policies and operational procedures of the HMO; engage in the coordinated practice of their profession and provide to enrollees of the HMO the health services under contract; share medical and other records, equipment, and professional, technical, and administrative staff of the HMO; and provide their professional services in accordance with a compensation arrangement, other than FFS, established by the HMO (including fee-for-time, retainer, or salary)

staff privileges incident—any act or omission arising from service by any insured as a member of an accreditation or credentialing committee or hearing panel of the named insured or by any person charged with executing the directives of such committee or panel while such person is acting within the scope of his duties in executing such directives, including an improper or unlawful denial or restriction of the claimant's staff privileges or wrongful failure to act upon the application or request for such privileges

standard benefit package—in managed cooperation, a package of medical services that must be provided to individuals, small businesses, and large businesses at competitive rates

standard class rate—*see SCR*

standard industry code—since various industries carry different incidents of injury and illness, this standard was established for the various sectors of the industry, as differentiators of health care costs based on experience

standard insurance—insurance written on the basis of regular morbidity underwriting assumptions used by an insurance company and issued at normal rates

standard prescriber identification number—*see SPIN*

standard reports—most management information system software contains standard reports, as opposed to customized ad hoc reports, which are generated to assist management in evaluating performance of providers, claims experience, or learning the characteristics of enrolled membership

standardized taxonomy—use of common standardized definitions, criteria, terminology, and data elements for treatment processes, outcomes, data collection and electronic transmission with the goal of saving much time, effort, and misunderstanding in communicating these elements; the health care industry is moving toward standards, after efforts led by NCQA, Health Outcomes Institute, HEDIS, the American Health Information Management Association, and others, but has not yet achieved standardized taxonomy

standards of performance—*see performance standard*

standing orders—the standardization of physician orders for procedures, tests, medications, and supplies for particular types of diagnosis treatment, or surgical procedures; created from clinical studies of best practices and are often modified within a hospital when initially obtained from an outside source; result in reduced costs if physicians have an incentive to use them

Stark I—effective January 1992 from the 1989 OBRA (42 U.S.C., 1395nn), precluding patient self-referrals by a physician to an entity of financial interest to the physician or relative, such as a clinical laboratory; formally called the Ethics in Patient Referrals Act and contains several exceptions to referral relationships or purposes; *see also self-referral restriction*

Stark II—effective August 1993 as strengthened restrictions of Stark I, further precluding patient referrals to an expanded list of health care services by a physician having financial interest in the referral entity

state action immunity—a state doctrine that provides exemption from federal antitrust review, assuming that joint ventures or mergers can meet the criteria of being able to defend the reason for reduced competition within a defined market, and undergo active review in the exempted area for market impact; some laws also call for a test to ensure that benefits outweigh the decreased competition, and annual progress reports; *see also COPA law*

statement of individual loss—many agreements call for the plan to submit a report to the reinsurer for any patient who exceeds the stop loss, for example any member who reaches $100,000 in allowable expenses; this statement includes the patient's personal information, nature of illness, payment calculations, and any amounts recovered from other insurance

stop loss or stop loss insurance—insurance that is designed to stop the loss, or limit risk exposure beyond a stated amount, for either the catastrophic loss of individual patients, or group claims; stop loss insurance is sought by nearly any entity that

accepts risk, and true to standard insurance concepts—the more protection the higher the insurance cost—so a point of attachment to stop loss at $75,000 might cost $2.50 PMPM, whereas an attachment at $100,000 might cost $2.00; *see also point of attachment, and reinsurance*

strategic alliance—may be either any structure listed within the definition of hospital alliance, or structures that also include various components of physician groups, or an HMO or MCO together with a hospital alliance for the purpose of effectively competing in a market and obtaining managed care business; *see also hospital alliance*

strategic hospital alliance—*see hospital alliance*

structured settlement—a strategy used by risk managers, insurers, and health institution attorneys to reduce the overall cost of making the payment on a legal claim to a plaintiff, by essentially using the "present value of money" technique—instead of paying a lump sum, the full payment is deferred while an annuity is purchased for the plaintiff using compounded interest rates that provide a stream of future income, which exceeds the one lump sum; structured settlement brokers with third-party corporations can relieve hospitals of the responsibility of making future payments; *see also risk management*

subacute care—a relatively new health care setting that has grown as a result of providing reduced cost in comparison to traditional acute hospitalization, yet providing the medical and skilled nursing required for patients that need more than long-term care (LTC); comprehensive inpatient care designed for someone who has had an acute illness, injury, or exacerbation of a disease process; generally more intensive than traditional nursing facility care and less intensive than acute care, requiring daily to weekly recurrent patient assessment and review; *see also continuum of care, and LTC*

subcapitation—any capitation arrangement at a level subordinate to global capitation, such as a subcap between an IDS and primary care physicians, specialists, or ancillary services

submitted charge—the amount that a provider bills to an insurer or patient; the amount that was most often reimbursed to the provider under fee-for-service medicine before managed care reform; *see also FFS*

subrogation—within the context of third-party claims, subrogation occurs when an insurer is able to recover from the enrollee some or all of the payment from legal action

subscriber—*see member*

substance abuse—the abusive consumption of alcohol, drugs, or chemicals that threatens the mental, physical, or financial health of an individual or others

substandard insurance—insurance issued with an extra premium or special restriction to persons who do not qualify for insurance at standard rates

summary plan description—*see SPD*

supplemental benefits—disability insurance provisions that allow benefits to increase the monthly indemnity or to give a portion of the policy premium if a policy is kept in for 5 or 10 years, or the insured does not file any claims; *see also supplemental health services*

supplemental health services—the health services not described as basic health services, as defined in section 417.102(a) of the Code of Federal Regulation for federally qualified HMOs; *see also additional benefits to Medicare risk*

supplemental medical insurance—*see SMI*

supplier—a specific interpretation and distinction of a "provider" within Medicare policy language P.L. 93-641, which defines a supplier versus a provider, thereby determining reimbursement on a cost-related basis versus prospective or retrospective (section 1531(3) of the PHS Act): "a direct provider of health care (including a physician, dentist, nurse, podiatrist, or physician assistant) in that the individual's primary current activity is the provision of health care to individuals or the administration of facilities or institutions (including hospitals, long-term care facilities, outpatient facilities, and HMOs) in which such care is provided and, when required by state law, the individual has received professional training in the provision of such care or in such administration is licensed or certified for such provision or administration"; *see also provider*

surgery schedule—list of maximum amounts payable by an insurance policy for various types of surgery, with the amount based on the severity of the operation

surgi-center—*see ASC*

surplus—a description of the funds remaining relative to a risk product or arrangement for payout as bonus or retention, either at the level of an HMO, a hospital withhold pool, an IPA, medical group, pod-level entity or individual PCP under full personal capitation; *see also withhold pool*

sustainable growth adjustment—the proposed annual adjustment for Medicare that essentially levies adjustments based on what can be financially sustained according to certain market factors; would be based upon the sustainable growth rate (SGR) calculation, which would include components of the change in Medicare Economic Index (MEI), change in the gross domestic product, and volume growth of enrollment into managed care options for Medicare; *see also MEI, and SGR*

sustainable growth rate—*see SGR*

sustainable growth rate system—a proposed revision by Congress and the Administration in 1996 to the Volume Performance Standard, with the objective of creating an improved and more timely tool for updating the Medicare fee schedule—by using gross domestic product growth targets and shortening the two-year delay currently used for the conversion factor; *see also VPS*

system capitation model—the description for any type of global capitation arrangement between a payer and an IDN with vertical integration; the system may involve owned or employed physicians, which enables the system to attract fully capitated contracts and be at risk for the care, while avoiding some of the governance and decision-making complexities of the network capitation model; *see also global capitation, IDN, network capitation model, and partnership capitation model*

systems integration (information systems)—generally refers to the outsourcing of certain information systems tasks to a consultant, which may include customer support for users, operations, the design and development of system interface requirements and software, product and vendor selection, system testing and evaluation, modeling, software and/or hardware configuration and installation, project management, and other services

systems integrator—a firm that delivers the various services of systems integration; *see systems integration*

table of allowances—*see covered services*

table rates—*see age/sex factor*

tail policy or tail coverage—normally provided to cover incidents of medical risk that were incepted during the policy period but not reported until after the policy period ended; coverage provided to a physician who leaves a program to retire or join another plan

TAT—turnaround time; a standard metric that is used to define the time required to process a health-related transaction, such as a medical claim

tax exemption—in addition to having no requirement to pay federal income taxes, qualifying tax exempt health care institutions can raise charitable contributions that are deductible to donors up to 50% of their gross income; organizations must be operated solely for a stated exempt purpose

taxonomy standards—*see standardized taxonomy*

TEFRA—Tax Equity and Fiscal Responsibility Act of 1982; the federal law containing many significant provisions for managed care, such as Medicare risk for HMOs and CMPs contracting with HCFA; TEFRA mandated Medicare for full-time workers between 65 and 69, and created cost-per-case limits and incentive payments to hospitals that keep their costs below a target amount

telemarketing—a staff function that allows a provider or health plan to contact prospective customers by telephone to explain managed care covered services and benefits, comparing them to traditional fee-for-service medicine in such a way that will motivate patients to enroll with the provider or plan; normally performed by member services representatives, or other staff members that have been trained to understand health care benefits structure; Medicare telemarketing must be done within the limits of Medicare marketing prohibitions; *see also Medicare marketing prohibitions, and open enrollment period*

telemedicine—the ability to use centralized medical expertise to provide care to patients of rural areas, and for centralized physicians to speak and share images with rural doctors through two-way visual and audio networks that allow an electronic house call; telemedicine, such as teleradiology, precludes the rural patient's need for transportation to an urban area to receive care, and reduces other staff or equipment costs in rural areas, servicing nearly a third of today's rural hospitals

telephone follow-up—*see patient telemanagement*

telephone hotline or physician directory—*see physician referral service*

telephone triage system—a demand management or customer-oriented tool that allows patients to call by telephone to relate their problems or medical symptoms; by use of preapproved medical protocols, the triage operator is able to give advice, prescribe home remedies, or determine whether the patient should be seen within a given time period; telephone triage systems have achieved positive results by precluding unnecessary visits to the emergency room, or to a doctor's office—most current systems are designed to err on the side of inviting the patient to be seen (or calling a physician directly) rather than to risk missing a genuine medical problem; for-profit companies offer standard protocol for sale to providers, which are often backed up by telephone recording devices to record conversations for possible review later; *see also nurse hotline, nurse triage system, and pediatric hotline*

temporary disability insurance—insurance that covers off-the-job injury or sickness and is paid for by deductions from a person's paycheck; administered by state agency; also called unemployment compensation disability or state disability insurance

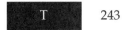

TennCare—an active Medicaid demonstration program within the state of Tennessee, which was designed to stop large losses due to Medicaid, beginning in 1994; reportedly saved $1 billion by summer of 1996 for 800,000 patients while expanding coverage to those previously uninsured, through allocating money to 12 private managed care organizations on a capitated basis of $1,214 in 1996; *see also capitation*

termination date—the ending date for eligibility of health care benefits because of expiration of the insurance period stated in the contract

termination without cause—this contracting clause provides for termination by either party without cause, subject to a reasonable notification period, as stated, such as 60, 90, or 120 days to minimize impact

tertiary care—health care treatment and services within a sophisticated specialty care setting that is approved under all requirements for tertiary care, serving as a referral and support alternative to primary and secondary care settings; *see also primary care, and secondary care*

third-party administrator—*see TPA*

third-party liability—exists if an entity is liable to pay the medical cost for injury, disease, or disability of a person hurt during the performance of his or her occupation and the injury is caused by an entity not connected with the employer; an increasingly significant consideration for recouping payment from over 20 possible sources that have been outlined in terms of sequential responsibility to pay by various state and federal laws, and the NAIC—beginning with the patient and extending through various group plan criteria, other individual and family insurance, Medicare, Medicare supplements, Program for the Handicapped, CHAMPUS/VA, or Maternal and Child Health or Indian Health Service, CHAMPUS supplements, and lastly Medicaid; *see also CHAMPUS, COB, NAIC, other party liability, and workers' compensation*

third-party payer—a public or private organization that pays for or underwrites coverage for health care expenses for another entity, usually an employer, such as Blue Cross and Blue Shield, Medicare, Medicaid, or commercial insurers; the individual enrollee generally pays a premium for coverage in all private and some public programs, then the organization pays bills on the patient's behalf, which are called third-party payments; also called third-party carrier

third-party payment—the third party is a payer or carrier that makes payment to a provider (the second party) on behalf of the patient (the first party)

third-party subrogation—*see subrogation*

time limit—a specified number of days in which a notice of claim or proof of a loss must be filed

time-phased plan—federally qualified HMOs may submit a time-phased plan to show how they will become operational, which may not extend for more than three years from the date of HCFA's determination, and specifies definite steps for meeting all the requirements of subparts B and C of CFR-42

total disability—the distinct level of disability beyond one year, due to a physical or mental illness or injury that makes an insured member unable to perform work for which they are qualified or educated, or limits the normal activities of a family member; eligibility for Medicare begins at the two-year point for disabled under 65 entitled under either the Social Security Act or the railroad retirement system

TPA—third-party administrator; any third-party entity that administers health plan entitlements and is supported by the infrastructure to process claims; a TPA does not underwrite the risk of a contract, but performs largely administrative functions that are supported by computer systems; as markets mature, many TPAs are looking to evolve into other lines of business, since HMOs and providers are becoming more able to perform the TPA primary mission

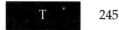

trade-off benefits—to provide substitute coverage for partial hospitalization or day treatment for inpatient care; such as outpatient rehabilitation for inpatient care on an ad hoc basis; although members have an absolute right to stated level of benefits, which cannot be decreased even if other benefits are added, trade-off benefits are sometime used without degradation

traditional indemnity plan—*see indemnity benefit contract*

traditional risk pool—*see hospital standard risk pool*

transitional bed—a bed with a lower associated daily cost than a standard inpatient bed, provided as a managed care strategy to provide an alternative setting that requires a lower medical staff support cost than acute care hospitalization, such as an observation unit, or skilled nursing facility; *see also SNF*

transitionally qualified HMO—an entity that operates a prepaid health care delivery system and that HCFA has determined meets the requirements of section 417.142(b) of CFR-42; a transitionally qualified HMO is considered a qualified HMO for the purpose of compliance by an employer with the requirements of section 1310 of the PHS Act and subpart E of CFR-42, which state that the employer must include the HMO in its health benefits plan so long as its qualification has not been revoked; these entities must meet operational requirements within 30 days of HCFA's determination as an operationally qualified HMO; *see also operational qualified HMO*

treatment episode—*see episode*

treatment facility—a generic reference to a hospital or clinic, or other category of health care entity, federal or nonfederal in which care is provided; or any mental health institution that meets the requirements established for treatment of substance abuse

treatment plan—an outline and format for reaching a treatment goal; *see also treatment protocols*

treatment protocols—a subset of medical protocols that serve as a reference for a physician, by outlining the recommended course of treatment for various conditions, to include follow-up requirements for the patient; *see also diagnosis protocols, medical protocols, and prevention protocols*

triage algorithm—an ordered set of medical decision tools, to assist a caregiver in making a decision about what care is needed, within a given time frame; the algorithm may be memorized for basic care decisions used in emergency medicine, or may be written or computerized for timely reference by a physician, nurse, technician, or EMT; *see also medical protocols*

triage hotline—*see telephone triage system*

TRICARE—the acronym given to the Department of Defense program of managed care, which uses a commercial HMO to supplement the health care services of the collective military treatment facilities; includes a triple option array of HMO (TRI-CARE Prime), PPO (TRICARE Extra), and indemnity type coverage (TRICARE standard, or traditional CHAMPUS); the coverage for the 50 states is divided into 12 regions, which are competitively bid

TRICARE Extra—the PPO-like coverage under the Department of Defense's TRICARE system, which offers no enrollment fee, lower copayment, no claims submissions by patients or balance billing to patients, and the choice of selecting a PCP who is not in the network

TRICARE Prime—the HMO-like coverage under the Department of Defense's TRICARE system, which offers no annual deductible, reduced copayments, access to Health Care Finder referral services, a primary care provider within the network of civilian participating providers or military providers, no balance billing, claims submissions, and point of service latitude for out-of-plan care; active duty military are automatically enrolled and receive a military PCP (and most of their care needs within the MTF); Medicare eligibles will be encouraged to enroll, if DoD is successful in obtaining reimbursement from

HCFA for money that otherwise would have been expended for Medicare of patients 65 and older

TRICARE Service Center—*see TSC*

TRICARE Standard—*see CHAMPUS*

triple option—the health care menu option that allows members to select from three choices for an HMO, PPO, or indemnity plan from one carrier; these selections carry incremental incentives for in-plan usage of physicians and network services, and corresponding disincentives of copays or deductibles; *see also HMO, PPO, and out-of-network*

trust fund—*see Medicare trust fund*

TSC—TRICARE Service Center; a staff function serving the Department of Defense military treatment facilities (MTFs) through contractor staffing from the insurer (or Managed Care Support Contractor), federal service staffing, or both, colocated with the MTF; the TSC provides member services support, claims assistance, and normally is staffed with a Health Care Finder, Health Benefits Advisor, and a combination of nursing and clerical support staff, depending upon the size of the supported MTF

turfing—transferring the sickest, high-cost patients to other physicians so the transferring provider appears to be a low utilizer

turnaround time—*see TAT*

two-way exclusives—a contract arrangement that guarantees that an insurer will use only one provider, and the provider will only contract with the insurer as a closed panel; *see also closed panel, and exclusivity*

UB-92—Uniform Billing Code of 1992, a revised version of the UB-82, a federal directive requiring a hospital to follow specific billing procedures, with an itemized invoice of medical services that were provided, with the corresponding charges; the UB-92 covers only the hospital or institutional charges, versus the HCFA 1500, which covers noninstitutional charges; *see also HCFA 1500*

UCR—usual, customary, and reasonable; *see reasonable and customary charge*

ultimate net loss—the total amount that the insured shall become legally obligated to pay as damages, whether actually expended or payable, either by actual adjudication or settlement arising with respect to each medical incident as respects the contract portion of Professional Liability (such as liability limits stated at $21,000,000 for each medical incident or an aggregate of $23,000,000) or General Liability (such as $21,000,000 for each occurrence or $23,000,000 for aggregate)

UM—utilization management; the process of evaluating the necessity, appropriateness, and efficiency of health care services; a review coordinator or medical director gathers information about the proposed hospitalization, service, or procedure from the patient and/or provider, then determines whether it meets established guidelines and criteria, which may be written or automated protocols approved by the organization; a provider or IDN that proves it is skilled in UM may negotiate more advantageous pricing, if UM is normally performed by the HMO but could be more effectively passed downward at a savings to the HMO

unbundling—the practice of a provider billing for multiple components of service that were previously included in a single fee; for example, billing the dressings and instruments for a minor procedure in addition to the procedure itself; unbundling is prohibited; billing under Medicare Part B for nonphysician services to hospital inpatients furnished to the hospital by an outside supplier or another provider; also called itemizing, a la carte medicine, fragmented billing, or exploded billing

underwriting—to bear risk for some potential loss; a review or statistical analysis of an individual or group profile to determine whether or not coverage should be given, and at what rate; the process of calculating the prospective data needed for appropriate pricing, risk assessment, and administrative feasibility

unified insurance—coverage by health insurance by a single policy

Uniform Bill 1992—*see UB-92*

uniformed services treatment facility—*see USTF*

unit cost risk pool—*see physician unit cost hospital pool*

universal access—a condition of a standard health benefits package so all individuals in the United States could have access to health care by 1999; made a central theme by discussions surrounding the 1992 U.S. presidential elections, and initially made part of the law in 1993 before reversal in 1995

unregulated provider entities—in the sense that the federal qualification procedures for HMOs involve regulations regarding financial strength, marketing capabilities, and systems, it may be said that other managed care entities that are allowed to assume risk are not held to a similar level of regulation; in August of 1995 the NAIC issued a memo to state regulators to ensure that all existing regulations were applied; meanwhile, attention was drawn to other aspects of regulation; *see also CLEAR, federal qualification, NAIC, PHO, and PSN*

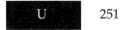

unusual or infrequently used services—those health services that are projected to involve fewer than 1% of the encounters per year for the entire HMO enrollment; or those health services the provision of which, given the enrollment projection of the HMO and generally accepted staffing patterns, is projected will require less than 0.25 full time equivalent (FTE) health professionals

upcoding—*see coding creep*

UR—utilization review; the evaluation of medical necessity, and efficiency or quality of health care services, either prospectively, concurrently, or retrospectively; contrasted with utilization management in that UR is more limited to the physician's diagnosis, treatment, and billing amount, whereas UM addresses the wider program requirements; *see also CM, discharge planning, and UM*

URAC—Utilization Review Accreditation Commission; chartered as an independent organization in 1990 to accredit and advance national standards in utilization and quality management programs; diverse board membership represents managed care, providers, public, and regulators' interests; has a relatively new focus toward expanding its role in accrediting noncapitated provider networks that pay providers based on either a fee schedule, discounted FFS, or DRG basis

urgent care center—a care facility providing immediate, but non-emergent care for minor illness or injury, allowing ambulatory walk-in service that may be either extended hour or 24-hour service; these facilities had their genesis in managed care principles to provide timely access to care that was less costly than emergency room settings

urgently needed services—this HCFA definition includes basically the blended contents of "covered services" and "out-of-area" emergencies; covered services required in order to prevent serious deterioration of an enrollee's health that results from an unforeseen illness or injury if the enrollee is temporarily absent from the HMO or CMP geographic area

urgi-center—*see urgent care center*

URO—utilization review organization; contracts with an integrated delivery network or managed care organization to perform utilization review; *see also UR*

U.S. Department of Health and Human Services—*see HHS*

U.S. per capita cost—*see USPCC*

U.S. per capita incurred cost—*see USPCC*

USPCC—U.S. per capita cost; the Medicare risk contract reimbursement rate based on three years of Medicare historical spending data that separates Parts A and B for the aged, disabled, and end stage renal disease; also adjusted for geographical AAPCC; includes intermediary or carrier administrative costs incurred by Medicare, as determined on an accrual basis; *see also AAPCC, and ESRD*

USTF—uniformed services treatment facility; includes all military treatment facilities (MTFs) and the former Public Health Service hospitals that are now called USTFs, which stands for Uniformed Services Treatment Facilities; USTFs are located in Baltimore, MD; Boston, MA; Seattle, WA; Portland, OR; Cleveland, OH; Houston, Galveston, Port Arthur, and Nassau Bay, TX; and Staten Island, NY; *see also MTF*

usual, customary, and reasonable—*see reasonable and customary charge*

uterine monitoring—the use of medical equipment in the home of pregnant women at high risk for preterm delivery, for uterine monitoring of labor contractions, and hopefully prolonging the onset of preterm delivery; used by many providers so that neonates are allowed to develop toward full term, with improved health, and less need of expensive medical care and Neonatal Intensive Care Unit charges; used in conjunction with patient education and daily nurse contact, versus instructing the patient how to detect early contractions through self-palpations

utilization—the use of health care services and supplies by an enrolled member or a group, which has become the focus of the managed care discipline, to ensure the medical necessity and appropriateness of all expenses; typically measured in areas of admissions per thousand patients enrolled, visits per thousand, or hospital bed days per thousand; *see also UM*

utilization management—*see UM*

utilization review—*see UR*

Utilization Review Accreditation Commission—*see URAC*

utilization review organization—*see URO*

V

V codes—a classification of ICD–9–CM coding to identify health care encounters for reasons other than illness or injury and to identify patients whose injury or illness is influenced by special circumstances or problems

VA disability program—a program for honorably discharged veterans who file claim for a service-connected disability

validation—verification of DRG assignment by finding that the diagnostic and procedural information is substantiated by the patient chart documentation

variable capitation–absolute scale—an incentive payment mechanism for physicians, using a corridor, such as 90%–130% of projected PMPM based on reduced utilization costs, with a monthly prospective adjustment of past performance, measuring performance on an established scale for all physicians (versus comparing peer performance as in variable capitation on a relative scale)

variable capitation–relative scale—an incentive payment mechanism for physicians, using a tiered range, such as 90%–130% of projected PMPM based on reduced utilization costs, with a monthly prospective adjustment of past performance, measuring performance on a scale that is relative to peers (versus an established scale for all physicians in variable capitation on an absolute scale)

variable cost risk pool—*see hospital variable cost risk pool*

vertical consolidation—the legal reference to vertical integration of health entities that have a relationship of supplier and customer; when these entities consolidate, they cause the elimination of a competitor or even a potential rival; closing access to a customer market by a rival or creating a market entry barrier; *see also antitrust laws, and vertical integration*

vertical integration—the connecting of dissimilar or other than strictly horizontal entities such as an HMO, hospitals, physician practices, PPO, or PHO into one care system from parts that used to exist as a supplier–customer relationship; linked to enhance coordination and value to patient care and support, while aiding proper utilization by the system; may be formed through joint ventures, mergers or acquisitions, new service development, or meaningful affiliations; also called full-service integration; *see also continuum of care, and horizontal integration*

vicarious liability—*see respondent superior*

virtual health care evolution—the sequential evolution of retail health care systems, depending on the particular market, in which the most recent transitions have normally progressed from direct contracting, to HIPCs and purchasing alliances, to the virtual care system model; *see also care system model, direct contracting, HIPC, and purchasing alliance*

virtual health care system—*see care system model*

vision carve out—managed care as a capitation reimbursement arrangement for eye care, which is a carve out segment of the PMPM or contract pricing; services may be as limited as an annual eye exam or as extensive as ASO claims services or volume discounts on lenses, contacts, custom tinting, and even on-site QA support for providers; some arrangements may require that ophthalmologists be participating providers if ophthalmology services are included in the coverage; *see also ASO*

visit rates per thousand—a utilization measurement unit that quantifies the annual use of noninstitutional providers, in terms of the number of visits to providers in a year per each thousand covered lives

VISN—veterans integrated service network; the recent streamlining goal of the Department of Veterans Affairs to reshape

how the VA delivers care; involves a rightsizing of the 172 hospitals and 530 other health care facilities, with more than 200,000 employees into 22 VISNs; planning and budget authority goes to network directors, not hospital administrators

voice response system—a unit that allows a customer to call in by telephone, and give instructions to a computer by speaking or by pressing digits on the phone; the input may be used in multiple health care applications to reduce costs, direct the caller to the appropriate office without use of an operator, and avoid other shortfalls of speaking with staff during certain limited business hours, such as pharmacy refill call-in systems, telephone appointments, or HMO member services customer support; may be part of an overall integrated call management system, to include call screen transfer capability; *see also call screen transfer capability, integrated call management, and open information systems architecture*

volume and intensity of service—a measurement of the quantity of health services per member, which includes the number of services and the complexity of the services rendered

volume offset—the health care utilization change in behavior, in terms of the number and mix of medical services that is projected to occur in response to a change in pricing

volume performance standard—*see VPS*

voluntary disability insurance—an option for disability insurance, versus a state-affiliated and mandated plan, wherein the majority of employees of an employer voluntarily consent to be covered by an insured or self-insured disability insurance plan

volunteer—any person whose services or labor are uncompensated from any source and whose activities are directed or supervised by, and for the benefit of, the named insured

voucher program—sometimes used to describe proposed managed care initiatives at the federal level that involve giving each person a coupon that would be valid for a given amount of health care or health care insurance, with the understanding that they would be responsible to find their own health care or insurance; also used to describe a fixed level of benefit within an employer voucher system that allows employees to select a provider, with or without using an HMO

VPS—volume performance standard system; a mechanism to adjust fee schedule updates for Medicare based on comparing annual cost increases to previously determined rates of increase; the desired growth rate for spending on Medicare Part B physician services, which is set each year by Congress after analysis by the Physician Payment Review Commission; *see also PPRC*

W

waiting period—the amount of time a person must wait from the date of entry into an eligible class, or from application for coverage to the date the insurance becomes effective

waiver of premium—an employee does not have to pay any premiums while disabled, if the policy contains this provision

WEDI—Workgroup for Electronic Data Interchange; a workgroup begun by the Secretary of HHS in 1991 as a means toward developing standards and recommendations to enhance the transmission of electronic health data

wellness program—any of a growing number of health education programs, directed toward healthier employees and reducing health care costs, which may include in-house or outside source expertise to assist with education, or to encourage exercise and other activities; data are important to form policies that best impact health status; *see also health promotion*

wholesale hospital marketing—a strategy of marketing to an insurer, from the perspective of a hospital or provider network, versus retail marketing directly to employers or patients; as managed care markets mature (and possibly aided by upcoming legislation for Provider Sponsored Networks), it is likely that hospital systems currently providing health care through wholesale arrangements will shift their emphasis toward retail arrangements in order to be able to profit from a larger portion of risk capitation; *see also broad panel health plan, exclusivity, PSN, and retail hospital marketing*

wholesale or wholesale HMO—commonly used to describe the market position of an IDS that is not willing or able to perform as an HMO in a retail sense, because it either does not possess a license or capital, or is not compelled by its mission to become a retail HMO; *see also retail HMO*

wireless technology—recent Radio Frequency (RF) architecture that transmits signals from remote, lightweight workstations to the wireless local area network (LAN) in such a way that health-related work processes can be reengineered toward greater mobility with an improved focus on the patient, such as bedside patient registration; *see also LAN*

withhold or withhold pool—*see PCR*

Work Relative Value—*see WRV*

workers' compensation—a program that provides liability insurance for the employer and benefits to the employees in the case of job-related injury, with added consideration for family members of employees who are killed in the line of duty; the premium is paid by the employer; rehabilitation entities attempt to reduce health care costs and the costs of lost employment value by speeding recovery and return to work

Workgroup for Electronic Data Interchange—*see WEDI*

World Wide Web services—*see on-line services*

wraparound coverage—*see wraparound plan*

wraparound plan—health plan coverage for copays and deductibles not covered under an enrollee's primary plan—often used in Medicare references; another use of this term with CHAMPUS TRICARE contracting with HMOs defines the HMO's responsibility to provide care or administrative support for those needs that go beyond the government's capability within the uniformed services treatment system; *see also copayment, deductible, Medigap policy, and TRICARE*

WRV—Work Relative Value; the average amount of work applied by the provider for a particular type of medical service; one of the three factors used within the Relative Value Scale that assigns weights to each medical service (and the payment appropriate for each weight); *see also RVS*

Z

zero premium—in some Medicare marketplaces, there is a practice of not charging any added monthly premium to what is already paid for coverage of Part B—versus the practice of an HMO getting a monthly premium in addition to what is paid to the federal government by the patient; as markets become more aggressive and a precedent is set by one HMO to accept zero premium, it quickly becomes the standard for that market

Pass This Order Form Along to a Colleague or Order a Copy for a Friend Today!

For faster service or to inquire about discounts for bulk orders, call
1-800-638-8437

Newly revised with more than 1,100 terms!

Publication date: April 1998, ISBN 0-8342-1144-0, Order #11440, 288 pages, 5 1/2 × 8 1/2 paperback, $19.95

30-Day, Risk-Free Reply Card

/ /   YES! I want to improve my practice with proven tools for greater efficiency. Please send me *The Managed Health Care Dictionary, Second Edition* [#11440, $19.95] for 30 days at no risk.

Check One:
/ /   Payment enclosed.
/ /   Bill my institution. Purchase order must be attached.
/ /   Bill me.

State sales tax, plus 8.5% postage and handling are additional. Aspen pays postage and handling on prepaid orders, and a full refund will be issued if you are not completely satisfied.

Signature _____

Daytime phone (____)_____

Name _____

Title _____

Organization_____

Address_____

_____

City, State, Zip _____

CB202